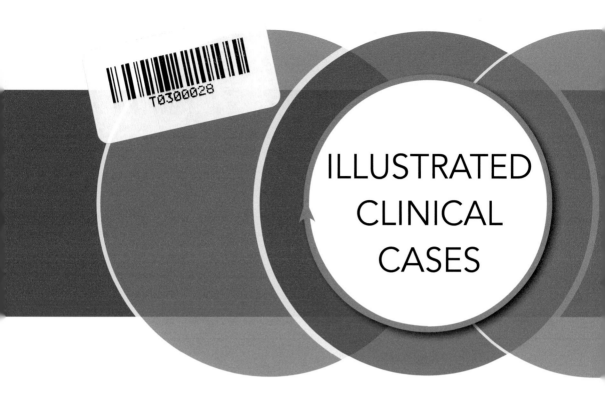

ILLUSTRATED CLINICAL CASES

Vascular Surgery

Providing real-world case examples and realistic mock examples of vascular surgery emergencies and clinical scenarios, this illustrated text supports trainees and residents in their daily clinical practice. However, the focus on senior decision-making and complex clinical management scenarios will also help trainees prepare for the FRCS (Vasc) and other specialist Vascular Surgery exams.

Indeed, making efficient and appropriate clinical decisions is one of the most important and challenging parts of postgraduate vascular surgical training. These realistic cases will teach trainee vascular surgeons to develop their diagnostic and management skills, expand their experience, and ultimately should empower them to form more advanced clinical management plans that reflect higher level thinking.

A broad range of clinical conditions are covered to ensure that the trainee vascular surgeon can respond with confidence when presented with difficult new case scenarios.

Illustrated Clinical Cases

About the Series

Each book of the *Illustrated Clinical Cases* series covers a specialized area of medicine, with clinical case scenarios and some challenging questions, followed by reasoned answers. The cases are presented randomly, as in real life, and are supported by superb diagrams and photographs of the highest quality. *Illustrated Clinical Cases* series titles are an invaluable text for both trainees and more established doctors in continuing professional development.

ENT Medicine and Surgery
Illustrated Clinical Cases
Simon Kinglsey Wickham Lloyd, Manohar Bance, Jayesh Doshi

Clinical Haematology, Second Edition
Illustrated Clinical Cases
Atul Bhanu Mehta, Keith Gomez

Dermatology
Illustrated Clinical Cases
William W. Huang, Steven R. Feldman, Christine S. Ahn, Robin S. Lewallen

Diagnosis of Non-accidental Injury
Illustrated Clinical Cases
Vincent J. Palusci, Dena Nazer, Patricia Brennan

Anaesthesia
Illustrated Clinical Cases
Magnus Garrioch, Bosseau Murray

Thoracic Imaging, Second Edition
Illustrated Clinical Cases
Sue Copley, David M. Hansell, Jeffrey P. Kanne

Cardiac Imaging
Illustrated Clinical Cases
Shahid Hussain, Jonathan Panting, Jun Kiat Teoh

Vascular Surgery
Illustrated Clinical Cases
James Michael Forsyth

For more information about this series please visit: https://www.crcpress.com/Illustrated-Clinical-Cases/book-series/CRCILLCLICAS

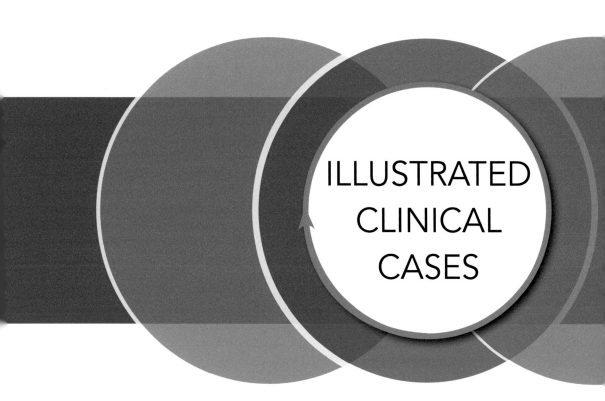

ILLUSTRATED
CLINICAL
CASES

Vascular Surgery

JAMES MICHAEL FORSYTH

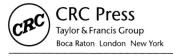

CRC Press
Taylor & Francis Group
Boca Raton London New York

CRC Press is an imprint of the
Taylor & Francis Group, an **informa** business

Designed cover image: Author's own image

First edition published 2025
by CRC Press
2385 NW Executive Center Drive, Suite 320, Boca Raton, FL 33431

and by CRC Press
4 Park Square, Milton Park, Abingdon, Oxon, OX14 4RN

CRC Press is an imprint of Taylor & Francis Group, LLC

© 2025 James Michael Forsyth

ISBN: 9781032804828 (hbk)
ISBN: 9781032804811 (pbk)
ISBN: 9781003497042 (ebk)

DOI: 10.1201/9781003497042

Typeset in Minion
by Deanta Global Publishing Services, Chennai, India

I dedicate this book to my parents John and Linda,
and my three sisters Aimee, Lucy, and Natalie

CONTENTS

HOW THIS BOOK IS SUPPOSED TO WORK

There are many vascular surgery resources out there:

- Textbooks
- Journal papers
- Guidelines
- Podcasts
- Videos
- Conferences

This book does not claim to be authoritative, nor does it claim to be the source of all wisdom, nor does it claim to be of equal value to any of the above. It is my hope that this book will be seen and interpreted somewhat differently. I want this book to be seen as a ***first-person experience***, but also an ***experience of walking a trodden path that many unseen vascular surgeons have walked before.*** As I write this opening text, I picture an enthusiastic young traveller who is trying to seek the safest route to the top of a dangerous mountain. There are a number of paths one could take, and there are many forks in the path as you progress with different subsequent paths to follow. It may be raining or snowing or sunny. One may have a compass and a map. One may be alone. One may be with friendly and experienced company.

I recall a few occasions in the past when I have climbed some relatively small mountains, and at various points these journeys have been extremely isolated. I have found myself looking around and realising that there is almost nobody here. It has felt lonely. It has felt cold. I have felt like I must be the only person who has ever climbed this mountain or walked this path. However, these superficial reflections are quickly met with an acceptance of reality. The truth is that many men and women have trodden these paths before me, and that is often why the path is so visible. There does come some added comfort from knowing that despite how big and jagged and dangerous and lonely some mountains may appear, others have been where you and I are now, they have followed similar paths to you and I, and they have safely made it to the top of the mountain.

The cases that I include in this book represent a very brief and discrete snapshot into my own brief journey along the vascular surgery mountain path. Some of the cases are descriptions of my own direct experiences, others are drawn from indirect lessons learnt, others are drawn from certain truths about vascular surgery which I picked up along the way. Certain cases have been fabricated and are designed to represent deliberate worse case scenarios, but they still draw out real-world lessons and contain a lot of truth within them.

A famous saying is this: "*The map is not the territory.*" Along my vascular surgery journey I have had the benefit of knowing guidelines and evidence and other surgeons' wisdom and experience and multidisciplinary team meeting (MDT) recommendations … but in my opinion this represents the **MAP**. Much of the challenge for me as a consultant has not been understanding how to read the **MAP**, but instead learning how to actually navigate through the real-world **TERRITORY**.

I endeavour therefore to provide the reader with cases that mainly focus on placing **YOU** within the confines of the real world. I wish to force upon you the reader the **TERRITORY,** and see how you navigate your way through it. I will give you various options along the way, but for the sake of ease and transparency I will provide some *not no subtle clues* as to what I believe the correct choices are. I will also display the path that actually has been trodden before so that if you encounter similar clinical cases or challenges in the future, it will hopefully help you to make forward progress along the correct routes (*and similarly avoid the more dangerous routes*).

It must be emphasised that because this book is about **TERRITORY** (*and not the MAP*) the focus will not be on evidence or guidelines. Much of that can be learnt from other vascular surgery educational resources. Instead, this book will focus on the following:

- Pragmatism (*i.e. choosing viable options that apply themselves to the actual clinical context*)
- Common sense (*i.e. doing what most other sensible vascular surgeons would do*)
- Basic principles (*e.g. proximal control, distal control, then attack the injury, etc.*)
- Dealing with relatively challenging cases (*i.e. the night on the mountain when you are cold and tired with poor visibility and difficult choices ahead*)
- Finding your way out of sticky spots and/or not getting yourself into sticky spots in the first place

Finally, this book represents my opinions. My opinions may be different to other peoples' opinions. This book is not gospel, and as such it should not be treated as such. If there are things of value within it, take it for yourself. If there are things which are not of value, ignore them.

James Michael Forsyth

You are the vascular surgeon on-call in a busy tertiary centre. It is 8 pm. You are alerted to a "code red" trauma call that is imminently about to descend upon A&E resus. You are informed that a 20-year-old male has been involved in a high-speed road traffic accident. The patient was in the front seat in a car travelling at around 60 mph. He was wearing a seat belt . His car collided with another car that was travelling at around 60 mph. Both cars were wrecked and the drivers of both vehicles died on scene. This patient is reported to be *verging* on haemodynamic instability, and he also had a low GCS on scene (8/15). The paramedics subsequently intubated him on scene and then brought him straight to A&E.

Primary survey information:

- *Airway* – intubated and ventilated. No immediate airway concerns.
- *Breathing* – air entry bilaterally with some crepitations mainly on the right side. No obvious flail chest.
- *Circulation* – heart rate now is 98. Blood pressure 104/64 mmHg. Capillary refill time centrally and peripherally is 2 seconds. Upper and lower limb pulses are all palpable. Abdomen appears soft and non-distended. No obvious femoral fractures. No obvious pelvic fracture.
- *Disability* – GCS is around 8. Pupils reactive and not dilated. Blood glucose is normal.
- *Exposure* – seat belt sign across chest. No external blood around the patient. Nil else on external examination.

What is your immediate management plan?

  A FAST scan.
  B Large bore IV access in both antecubital fossa and then urgent CT trauma series.
  C Large bore IV access via right internal jugular vein and FAST scan.
  D Theatre for immediate diagnostic +/– therapeutic laparotomy.
✓ E Pelvic binder, large bore IV access in both antecubital fossa and then urgent CT trauma series.

The patient goes for a full CT trauma scan. What do you make of the injuries shown in the images in Figure 1.1?

  A Type A aortic dissection and mediastinal haematoma.
  B Cardiac tamponade.
  C Massive right haemopneumothorax.
✓ D Aortic transection/large aortic pseudoaneurysm and mediastinal haematoma with evidence of right pulmonary contusion.
  E Oesophageal rupture into right chest.

How would you interpret this CT report? What would be your management plan?

- CT chest abdomen pelvis conclusion: *"Traumatic aortic injury. Liver lacerations with no active haemorrhage. Fractured right first second and third ribs with associated right-sided pneumothorax and pulmonary contusions. Right sided pelvic and sacral fractures with disruption of the pubic synthesis."*
- CT head: *"Features of intra-cranial injury with small volume subarachnoid and intra-ventricular haemorrhage. Potential features of axonal injury, clinical correlation required."*

DOI: 10.1201/9781003497042-1

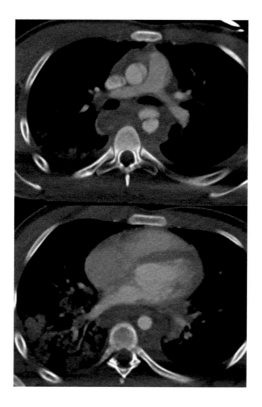

Figure 1.1

   A Laparotomy, liver packing, and pelvic packing.
   B Open repair of descending thoracic aorta via left posterolateral thoracotomy and inter-position tube graft repair (*"clamp-and-sew" approach*).
✓ C Emergency thoracic aortic stent insertion (TEVAR).
   D Urgent referral to neurosurgery for decompressive craniotomy.
   E ICU admission for medical optimisation, repeat CT aorta in 48 hours, followed by TEVAR if pseudoaneurysm is increasing in size.

You decide that the patient's most pressing injury is the aortic injury. Your plan is for an urgent TEVAR. You discuss the case with the consultant vascular interventional radiologist on-call, who is concerned that this patient's femoral and iliac arteries are a bit small and that the aorta is also quite small. Essentially, they are concerned that they may not be able to get an emergency thoracic aortic stent up (*from below*), and even if they were able to, the stent may be "too big" for the thoracic aorta. How would you respond to these concerns (*please review Figure 1.2 in conjunction with answering this question*).

   A Proceed immediately to thoracotomy and open surgical repair of the aortic injury.
   B Right axillo/subclavian artery cutdown and TEVAR from above.
✓ C Just get the TEVAR in quickly via femoral access. If there is an ileofemoral artery injury this can be fixed. Stopping the patient's aorta from rupturing is the current priority, and speed is of the essence. The aorta is also most likely vasoconstricted because the patient is shocked.
   D Laparotomy and direct infra-renal aortic exposure to allow TEVAR access.
   E Retroperitoneal exposure of iliac artery and iliac conduit creation to allow TEVAR access.

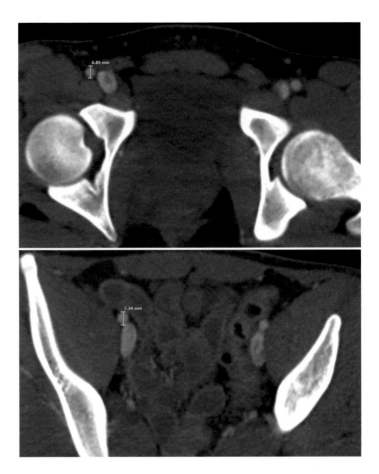

Figure 1.2

The plan is for an emergency TEVAR via femoral access. The patient's family arrive in A&E and want a full update. They want to know what is happening, what the predicted outcome is going to be, if there is a head injury, how bad is the head injury, what procedure is being planned, where the patient will be post-procedure ... ??? What are you going to say to the family?

   A "Your son is in a critical condition. He has a life-threatening aortic injury and time is of the essence here. He needs a time-critical procedure to try and stop him bleeding to death. I cannot stay here and answer all your questions because he needs this procedure as soon as possible. I will update you afterwards. I have to go."

   B Ignore the family completely.

✓ C "Your son is in a critical condition. He has a life-threatening aortic injury and time is of the essence here. He needs a time-critical procedure to try and stop him bleeding to death. I cannot stay here and answer all your questions because he needs this procedure as soon as possible. I will update you afterwards. I have to go, but the A&E team can update you in further detail during the interim."

   D "Your son is in a critical condition. He was in a high-speed road traffic accident. He is in a critical condition. He has multiple injuries including a head injury, rib fractures, lung contusions, a major arterial injury that is life-threatening, a liver injury, and a pelvic fracture. He requires an urgent procedure to try and stop him bleeding to death. This requires puncturing the femoral artery with a needle, passing a wire up towards his chest, and deploying a stent to cover the area where his artery has been damaged. He will require surveillance scans after this. This procedure also carries risks such as bleeding, infection, neurovascular injury, worsening limb ischaemia, limb loss, and death. There is also a risk his head injury is severe and he may be left with significant neurological disabilities even if this procedure is successful. He may spend months in hospital being rehabilitated after this procedure. I can draw you a diagram to demonstrate how the TEVAR procedure works, and I can also show you the consent form 4 I have just completed. If you have further questions we can go into a A&E relatives room and I can spend another 20 minutes explaining things further?"

E "I cannot talk now, sorry. I will speak to you after the procedure, but I will ask the A&E team to answer any questions in the interim."

The A&E team have referred the patient to orthopaedics in regard to the pelvic fractures evident on CT. What ways are there to achieve initial pelvic stabilisation within this context? Choose from the options below:

A Pelvic binder.
B Urgent ex-fix in orthopaedic theatre.
✓ C Wrap ankles together using a bed sheet.
D Urgent pelvic open repair and internal fixation in orthopaedic theatre.
E Patient does not require any form of pelvic stabilisation at the moment.

The patient arrives in the interventional radiology suite. He quickly decompensates as he is positioned onto the table. His systolic blood pressure drops to 39 mmHg systolic. He looks pale. What are some potential explanations for this profound and sudden haemodynamic deterioration? What do you think has happened?

A Liver has ruptured and catastrophic intra-peritoneal bleeding.
B Massive pelvic haemorrhage.
✓ C Aortic rupture.
D Myocardial infarction.
E Cardiac tamponade.

The interventional radiologist asks you if there is time for Proglide access to the groin to allow minimally invasive closure of the femoral artery at the end of the TEVAR procedure. Which answer are you going to give?

✓ A There is no time. The patient has likely ruptured his aorta and is now peri-arrest. The TEVAR needs to be deployed immediately. Therefore forget about the Proglides … just get the TEVAR in and up as quickly as possible. The femoral artery can be directly repaired afterwards via an open surgical approach.
B There is plenty of time here, so please take your time. Everybody needs to relax. Please achieve Proglide access and then get the TEVAR in. You would rather avoid an open surgical cutdown to the femoral artery in this context so it seems reasonable to take a bit of extra time at the beginning.
C No time for TEVAR now. Proceed to thoracotomy in the interventional radiology suite.
D Do a rapid groin cutdown, expose the femoral artery, and allow direct femoral artery puncture.
E Abandon the procedure. The patient has now ruptured his aorta and the time window to salvage the situation has now passed.

Please review this TEVAR post-procedural image (Figure 1.3).

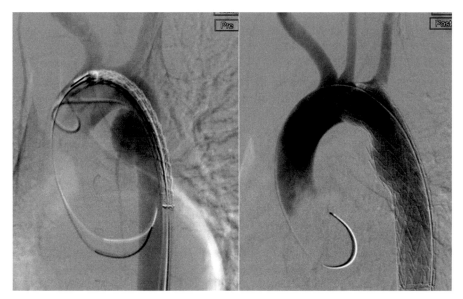

Figure 1.3   Successful TEVAR deployment.

The interventional radiologist did not use Proglides. You do a surgical cutdown and find that the CFA anterior wall is now quite "tattered" after removing the sheath. How would you repair the femoral artery?

    A Primary suture repair.
    B Bovine or Dacron patch repair.
✓ C Ipsilateral great saphenous vein (GSV) patch repair.
    D Contralateral great saphenous vein (GSV) patch repair.
    E CFA interposition graft repair using a prosthetic graft.

CASE REFLECTIONS

Severe descending thoracic aortic injuries like these (*basically an aortic transection*) are commonly associated with high-speed blunt trauma, particularly with high-speed road traffic accidents and co-existent seat belt use. Patients will often present with poly-trauma (*precisely because it is a blunt mechanism and the whole body takes a beating*), a seat belt sign is not uncommon, and patients will often complain of severe chest or back pain (*classically inter-scapular pain*).

You should therefore be cognisant of the fact that when you are presented with this type of vascular injury, it is **very likely** that you are going to have to manage other significant injuries at the same time. For example

- Pelvic fractures.
- Solid organ injuries (*classics would be spleen and/or liver*).
- Pulmonary contusions/rib fractures/flail chest/haemopneumothorax.
- Head injuries.
- Upper and lower limb fractures (*open or closed fractures with or without neurovascular compromise*).

Indeed, such other injuries may be quite impressive and cause some commotion/controversy amongst the other trauma team members. On occasion, it can be challenging to decide which injury is the most pressing problem. However, usually the "switched-on" vascular surgeon can make the right call quickly – **trust your instincts**.

Furthermore, you must maintain a high degree of caution in regard to this injury pattern, and here are some classic traps not to fall into.

TRAP 1

- Overestimating the degree of aortic injury. If you have a truly minor aortic injury then take a step back and survey the big picture. For example, a small dissection flap in the aorta that is not flow-limiting can almost certainly be observed with a plan for repeat imaging in a few days. In such an instance you should definitely not go pursuing an emergency TEVAR if the patient has got a ruptured spleen and a belly full of blood! Similarly, if the patient has a minor aortic injury and a large extradural haematoma with significant midline cerebral shift then guess what … the neurosurgeons should be going first!

TRAP 2

- Underestimating the degree of aortic injury and being distracted by other seemingly *impressive* but *far less life-threatening injuries*. For example, a very large aortic pseudoaneurysm and mediastinal haematoma is at an extremely high risk of rupture and death (*which clearly almost happened in this case*). In this context, a liver laceration that is not actively bleeding should not be pursued but instead managed conservatively. A relatively minor pelvic ring injury with no active pelvic bleeding should be temporarily managed conservatively with a straightforward simple means of pelvic stabilisation such as pelvic binding or wrapping the ankles together. An open wrist fracture with neurovascular compromise may well be managed quickly in A&E resus with reduction and back-slabbing … but certainly ***the wrist fracture is not going to kill the patient***. Therefore, do not sit idly by whilst the orthopaedic team takes the patient to theatre to fix the wrist because there is "neurovascular compromise" and simultaneously downgrade the lethal aortic injury. The last thing you want is to formally pursue less lethal injuries and fix them in theatre over the course of the next few hours, only to have the patient rupture their aorta 3 hours later and die.

TRAP 3

- Getting drawn into prolonged discussions with family members at the wrong time. The priority in the "code red" setting is to save the patient's life. The family should be *briefly updated* if time allows, but you do need to be assertive with family members and highlight to them that the time for detailed discussions must come later on (*after the initial life-saving interventions have been completed*). These large aortic pseudoaneurysms can rupture at any minute, and this time of "stability" whilst waiting for the TEVAR is the time to be getting blood available, maybe filling in a consent form 4, maybe wheeling the patient around the interventional radiology, etc.

TRAP 4

- Getting shunted into open aortic surgery because of "less than ideal" anatomical factors. To be frank, this situation is never going to be ideal. However, the gold standard approach for this pathology is now TEVAR. If the femoral arteries or iliac arteries are a bit small, then so be it. If the TEVAR will go up, then fair game. If the femoral/iliac access arteries definitely will not allow TEVAR access, then consider right axillosubclavian access. The notion of an iliac conduit in this author's opinion is largely academic – if you are putting an emergency TEVAR in a patient with a very large aortic pseudoaneurysm and mediastinal haematoma, then the argument can be made that you really don't have time to be doing an iliac conduit anyway. Similarly, within the context of a proposed thoracotomy, it is this author's opinion that this option is probably academic also. The time to be doing thoracotomies and sewing in an aortic graft is if the patient has arrested in front of you in A&E resus … however, if you find yourself doing this, you have almost certainly "missed the boat" and/or the "horse has already bolted." Even if the patient has not arrested, surely if someone has smashed up their entire body at a combined speed of 120 mph, already has pulmonary contusions and rib fractures and pelvic fractures and a severe head injury … opening their left chest is a pretty massive hit in addition to the above. The author of this case study recommends avoiding the "clamp-and-sew" approach if at all possible. ***If a TEVAR will go up, get it up quickly.***

TRAP 5

- Forgetting the possible consequences of TEVAR. Do not forget about the risk of spinal cord ischaemia, potentially a left posterior circulation stroke because of compromising the left vertebral artery, and also rarely left upper limb ischaemia. Maintain a decent systolic blood pressure, a decent haemoglobin, and decent oxygenation. Keep an eye on the left hand (*rarely you might have to do a left carotid-subclavian bypass*).

TRAP 6

- Naively expecting a globally positive outcome. These patients can have a pretty horrific overall trauma burden. You may have saved the patient's life by stopping the aorta from exploding… but the life they are now left with will be a reflection of what the rest of the trauma CT reported. Fortunately in this case the patient did survive, his left arm was not ischemic, his CFA repair was successful, and he had foot pulses afterwards. His TEVAR is positioned nicely on follow-up imaging, and he is making reassuring progress after input from the complex rehabilitation team.

TRAP 7

- Forgetting the femoral access complication. This does not specifically apply in this case because the femoral artery was repaired directly. However, as a general point of consideration, after any endovascular procedure via the femoral artery you should always examine the ipsilateral groin and confirm the distal pulse status. These patients can still get CFA dissections/EIA dissections, pseudoaneurysms, groin haematomas … the last thing you want is to save the patient's life and transfer them to ICU @ 11 pm, only to then have to take them back to theatre 6 hours later because they have an ischaemic leg.

EXPLANATION OF SOME OF MY ANSWERS TO THE QUESTIONS ABOVE

Pelvic Binder

- You cannot get access to the femoral arteries whilst a pelvic binder is on. Therefore, if you have a vascular emergency and need femoral access and the patient has a pelvic injury, just wrap the ankles together.

CFA Repair

- If you need to repair a femoral artery in an emergency damage control setting (*i.e. uncontrolled trauma setting*) then it is better to use autologous vein. Pragmatically in this case there was no deep venous injury therefore ipsilateral groin GSV was very

Vascular Surgery

easy to harvest and seemed to be the most expedient and sensible solution. GSV has increased resistance to infection. If this was an SFA trauma ischaemic limb context and you needed to do a full bypass, the correct examination answer however is to use contralateral GSV. Others would support using prosthetic material for a patch repair, which is not the wrong answer in the appropriate setting ... but putting prosthetic material into the groin of a young man is something I would rather avoid. A simple suture repair is always going to be ideal, but if it is already a small artery that has "tolerated" a large sheath and is now looking pretty tattered ... a primary suture repair is hopeful at best.

A 55-year-old male presents to the diabetic foot clinic with a new area of ulceration over his left 5th metatarsal head. It is probing down to underlying gritty bone and there are signs of minor soft tissue infection surrounding the ulcer and some overlying slough. The patient is also complaining of minor rest pain and night pain in the left forefoot, and occasionally he has to sleep with his left leg hanging out of bed. He has a good ipsilateral femoral pulse but nil pulses distally. He has monophasic ankle signals using the handheld Doppler. He has evidence of neuropathy. He also has a background of ischaemic heart disease and heart failure (*recent echocardiogram revealed a left ventricular ejection fraction of 30%*). The patient is also complaining of life-limiting intermittent calf claudication in his right leg and has only a right femoral pulse which is slightly reduced in volume compared to the left. He has no rest pain, night pain, or tissue loss in the right leg.

What is your working diagnosis?

✓ A Neuroischaemic left foot ulceration/chronic limb-threatening ischaemia.
  B Neuropathic left foot ulceration.
  C Pyoderma gangrenosum.
  D Mixed arteriovenous ulceration.
  E Necrotising fasciitis.

What is your management plan?

  A Best medical therapy, smoking cessation advice, toe pressure and WIfI staging, vein mapping, urgent CT angiogram lower limbs.
  B Best medical therapy, smoking cessation advice, vein mapping, urgent arterial duplex.
  C Best medical therapy, smoking cessation, vein mapping, urgent MR angiogram, toe pressure and WIfI staging.
✓ D Best medical therapy, smoking cessation, bone sampling from the base of ulcer (*for microscopy culture and sensitivity*), oral antibiotics for presumed osteomyelitis, offloading footwear, foot x-ray, vein mapping, arterial duplex +/− MRA/CTA.
  E Best medical therapy, smoking cessation, bone sampling from the base of ulcer (*for microscopy culture and sensitivity*), oral antibiotics for presumed osteomyelitis, offloading footwear, foot x-ray, vein mapping, straight to diagnostic angiogram +/− proceed.

His left hallux toe pressure is 34 mmHg. What is his WIfI stage?

  A 4 (1 2 2– high amputation risk, high potential benefit from revascularisation).
✓ B 4 (2 2 2– high amputation risk, high potential benefit from revascularisation).
  C 2 (1 1 1– low amputation risk, moderate potential benefit from revascularisation).
  D 4 (3 3 1– high amputation risk, high potential benefit from revascularisation).
  E 3 (1 2 1– moderate amputation risk, high potential benefit from revascularisation).

Please review Figure 2.1 to appreciate the microbiological and radiological context of the left 5th MT head "clinical" osteomyelitis.

DOI: 10.1201/9781003497042-2

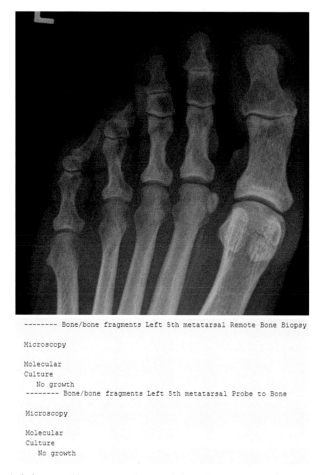

```
-------- Bone/bone fragments Left 5th metatarsal Remote Bone Biopsy

Microscopy

Molecular
Culture
   No growth
-------- Bone/bone fragments Left 5th metatarsal Probe to Bone

Microscopy

Molecular
Culture
   No growth
```

Figure 2.1 X-ray left foot and bone sample result for microscopy, culture, and sensitivity.

What is your interpretation of the x-ray and bone sample results?

   A Patient has radiological and microbiological osteomyelitis and requires 4–6 weeks of targeted antibiotics.

✓ B Patient does not have radiological or microbiological confirmation of osteomyelitis, but clinically does have osteomyelitis, so requires 4–6 weeks of empiric antibiotics.

   C Patient has radiological and clinical confirmation of osteomyelitis, but microbiology samples are negative so the patient does not require 4–6 weeks of antibiotics.

   D Patient does not have radiological, microbiological, or clinical signs of osteomyelitis, so should be treated with a shorter course of antibiotics for soft tissue infection alone.

   E Patient has radiological, clinical, and microbiological signs of osteomyelitis, so he requires 4–6 weeks of targeted antibiotics.

The patient ultimately has an MRA. What is your interpretation of Figure 2.2?

✓ A No inflow disease. Left short SFA occlusion with proximal AT, peroneal and PT stenoses but all three crural vessels patent distally. Right CFA significant stenosis with significant mid-right SFA stenosis.

   B Long left SFA occlusion with normal 3-vessel run-off. Right EIA severe stenotic disease and normal run-off on right.

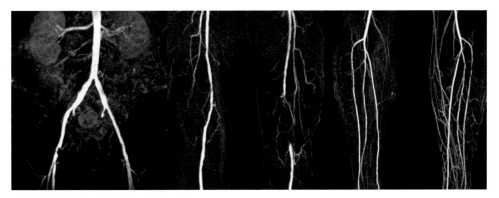

Figure 2.2   MRA lower limbs.

  C Significant left CFA and profunda origin disease, left severe SFA stenotic disease, diseased 3-vessel crural run-off. On the right side there is a short CFA occlusion with a short mid-SFA occlusion and diseased 2-vessel run-off via the AT and peroneal.

  D Small infra-renal AAA, left EIA minor stenotic disease, short left SFA occlusion, and normal 3-vessel run-off. Right CFA minor disease and normal run-off vessels.

  E Bilateral CIA origin stenotic disease, left SFA short occlusion, and diseased 3-vessel run-off. Right significant CFA disease and mid-SFA significant stenosis.

This is the left leg vein map result:

- GSV @ groin = 0.48 cm.
- GSV i@ mid-thigh = 0.38 cm.
- GSV @ knee level = 0.36 cm.
- GSV @ mid-calf = 0.37 cm.
- "Long, straight, compressible, no signs of thrombophlebitis, no venous reflux."

What would be your revascularisation plan for the left leg?

  A Left CFA endarterectomy, profundaplasty, and femoral to below-knee popliteal bypass using ipsilateral GSV.

  B Left SFA-AK popliteal bypass using PTFE with vein cuff.

  C Left iliac stenting, CFA endarterectomy, and fem-AT bypass using ipsilateral GSV.

✓ D Left antegrade angiogram with a view to SFA angioplasty +/– stenting +/– crural angioplasty.

  E Left femoral to above-knee popliteal artery bypass using contralateral GSV.

What would be your revascularisation plan for the right leg?

✓ A None. He does not have CLTI nor short distance claudication. This will be managed conservatively with best medical therapy, smoking cessation, and exercise therapy.

  B Right CFA endarterectomy.

  C Right CFA endarterectomy and downstream SFA angioplasty.

  D Right CFA endarterectomy and femoral to above-knee popliteal bypass using a prosthetic graft and a vein cuff.

  E Right CFA endarterectomy and femoral to BK popliteal artery bypass using prosthetic graft with a vein cuff.

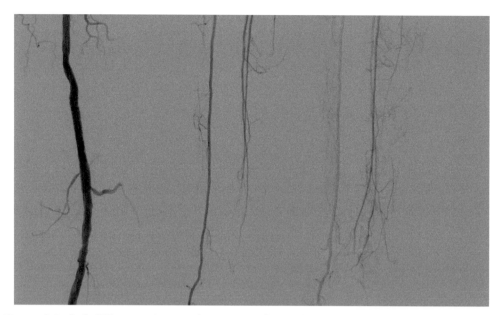

Figure 2.3 Left SFA angioplasty and stenting with crural vessel run-off views.

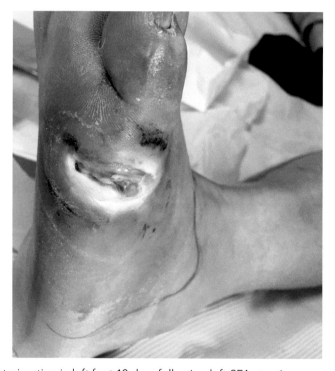

Figure 2.4 Deterioration in left foot 10 days following left SFA stenting.

This patient went for a left antegrade angiogram and ultimately had left SFA stenting with a good radiological result (see Figure 2.3). His right leg was managed conservatively. He was commenced on the VOYAGER regime following his angioplasty (aspirin 75 mg OD and rivaroxaban 2.5 mg BD). He was also commenced on atorvastatin 80 mg 0D aiming for an LDL of ≤1.4.

Ten days post-SFA stenting the patient re-presents with worsening clinical infection of the left foot. There is a small amount of pus expressed from the 5th MT head ulcer with exposed MTP joint at the base of the wound. There is erythema in the forefoot (see Figure 2.4). The patient is spiking temperatures with a heart rate of 104. The patient has a palpable popliteal and PT pulse with a hallux toe pressure of 67 mmHg (*although the left 5th toe looks slightly ischaemic*). What would your management plan be now?

  A Oral antibiotics and outpatient management.
  B Intravenous antibiotics alone.
✓ C Intravenous antibiotics and left 5th ray amputation.
  D Crural vessel angioplasty and intravenous antibiotics.
  E Crural vessel angioplasty, intravenous antibiotics, and left 5th ray amputation post-revascularisation.

CASE REFLECTIONS

This is a fairly standard patient for the diabetic foot clinic. The work-up is usually fairly standard also, especially if there is underlying peripheral arterial disease with tissue loss:

- Best medical therapy.
- Smoking cessation.
- Optimise diabetic control.
- Offloading footwear.
- If there is an ulcer does it probe to bone? Is there clinical evidence of osteomyelitis? If so, the usual pathway is bone sampling for microscopy, culture, and sensitivity and commence on appropriate empiric oral antibiotics (*often co-amoxiclav and amoxicillin in my current department*) while sensitivities await, and a foot x-ray.
- If there is an ulcer but it does not probe to bone and there is soft tissue infection, the treatment would usually be 2 weeks of oral flucloxacillin (*if not penicillin allergic*).
- The vascular work-up includes: assessing the lower limb pulse status, handheld Doppler signal assessment, toe pressure, and WIfI staging. After this if there is a femoral pulse the NICE and ESVS guidelines would support arterial duplex +/− vein mapping +/− cross-sectional imaging (MRA or CTA) – but only if you are planning revascularisation.
- If a patient had a popliteal pulse (*i.e. suspected crural vessel disease*) such a patient would likely go straight for an antegrade femoral angiogram +/− proceed. However, depending upon patient fitness and availability of autologous vein, the outcome would either be for a primary endovascular approach or to get some decent run-off imaging if a popliteal-distal bypass was being considered.

In this patient's case there were a few subtle areas of controversy. Should we treat for osteomyelitis even though the x-ray does not show obvious osteomyelitis and the bone samples were negative? In this specific case our DLS MDT supported on-going treatment for clinical osteomyelitis with empiric antibiotics because the clinical suspicion was high. In regard to the left leg revascularisation plan there is also potentially a further degree of controversy. This patient did have a 10 cm SFA occlusion with a decent ipsilateral GSV … surely there was an argument for a bypass? Well no … he was not that "fit" with an ejection fraction of 30% and ischaemic heart disease, it was a relatively short occlusion, and it looked extremely appetising for an endovascular first approach.

In essence, the work-up for this type of patient is fairly standard, but the decision-making in all cases can be nuanced and subjective and complex. There will always be a mixture of opinions on how best to manage diabetic foot patients. Perhaps this case further reflects the value of the DLS MDT and CLTI MDT. The other area of possible controversy is in regard to the right leg. Fair enough, the patient does have multi-level disease and is theoretically suitable for a right CFA endarterectomy +/− downstream SFA angioplasty. However, the priority at the moment is the left leg as this is the limb-threatening problem. The right leg is troubled by intermittent claudication, i.e. it is a life-limiting problem. There is evidence that patients with intermittent claudication who go for early revascularisation are at increased risk of major amputation in the long-term. Furthermore, one must prioritise the left leg and not get unnecessarily distracted by the right leg. In summary, although there are some areas of controversy, I believe that an endovascular first approach for the left leg was entirely reasonable, conservative management for the right leg was entirely reasonable, and treating the patient for clinical osteomyelitis was also entirely reasonable.

Finally, when the patient presented with worsening foot sepsis post-revascularisation with pus coming out of the foot (*i.e. the classic reperfusion sepsis*), clearly medical management had failed and the next logical step was a toe amputation. The old adage here would be: "Don't let the sun go down on a diabetic foot" and "pus in a diabetic foot equals theatre." In this case the left 5th ray amputation site did heal reasonably well. However, as can be seen on his angiographic images at the time of SFA stenting, there was residual crural vessel disease … and as such there is an argument in this case that further crural endovascular intervention may have been justified (*i.e. to achieve in-line flow via the AT perhaps although there was in-line flow to the foot via the PT*). Indeed, if there were further wound healing problems this would likely have triggered a further antegrade angiogram with a view to further crural angioplasty (*although his WIfI stage post SFA stenting and at the time of his worsening foot sepsis was 3- 2 0 2, which gave him a moderate amputation risk and very low potential benefit at the time of 5th ray amputation*). Ultimately, these are judgement calls … there is another argument here that "perfection is the enemy of good."

A 56-year-old male who is well known to the vascular surgery team re-presents with left foot rest pain, night pain, and tissue loss to his forefoot. He has had multiple endovascular procedures to his left leg already, left-sided toe amputations, and a failed bypass in the right leg that sadly resulted in a right above-knee amputation last year. He has additional extensive comorbidities: atrial flutter, metallic aortic valve replacement on warfarin, chronic kidney disease stage 3, heart failure, ischemic heart disease (NSTEMI 2021), type 2 diabetic mellitus on insulin, hypertension, iron deficiency anaemia, and vitamin D deficiency. He is an active smoker. On examination he has a decent ipsilateral left femoral pulse and no pulses distally. He has weak monophasic ankle signals with an unrecordable toe pressure. His left foot displays a punched out necrotic/ischaemic ulcer over the medial aspect of the 1st metatarsal head with no gross clinical infection. His left 5th toe has been previously amputated, but there is a similar small area of dry ischaemic ulceration over the remnant 5th metatarsal head. The left foot is Buerger's positive.

What is your interpretation of the MRA image (Figure 3.1)?

   A Long left SFA occlusion, BK popliteal is patent, and 2-vessel run-off via the AT and peroneal.

✓ B Long left SFA occlusion, BK popliteal is patent, 2-vessel run-off via the AT and peroneal, but the AT origin is possibly diseased, and the peroneal cuts off just above the ankle.

   C Left SFA stenotic disease, and decent 2-vessel run-off to the foot.

   D Significant left CFA disease, SFA stenotic disease, and decent 2-vessel run-off to the foot.

   E Left EIA disease, patent CFA, short SFA occlusion, and reconstitution in a diseased AT single-vessel run-off.

What is your interpretation of these previous angiographic images (*his last intervention 3 months ago before the recent MRA when he had diffuse SFA stenotic disease, see* Figure 3.2)?

   A Left SFA has been angioplastied. There is some AT origin disease, but the AT is otherwise patent down to the foot. The peroneal is patent down to the ankle.

✓ B Left SFA has been angioplastied. There is AT origin disease, but the AT is otherwise patent down to the foot. The peroneal is patent down to the ankle, when it collateralises and cross-fills to supply to heel.

   C The left SFA is patent and disease-free. There is minor disease of the AT origin.

   D The left SFA has been angioplastied and there is decent 2-vessel run-off via a disease-free AT and peroneal.

   E Patent and disease-free left SFA with severe 3-vessel disease below the knee.

What is your interpretation of this ipsilateral GSV vein map report from 3 months ago – around the time of his last left leg endovascular procedure (see Figure 3.3)?

   A This is a decent ipsilateral GSV in the thigh, but it is unsuitable below the knee.

   B This is a decent ipsilateral GSV for a below-knee popliteal bypass, but not for a distal (*AT or peroneal*) bypass.

   C The ipsilateral GSV is of decent quality for a distal bypass, but there is deep venous disease, so one should consider using the contralateral GSV.

✓ D The ipsilateral GSV appears to be of decent quality for a distal bypass.

   E This is a completely unreliable vein map report because the patient was examined supine.

DOI: 10.1201/9781003497042-3

Figure 3.1 MRA lower limbs.

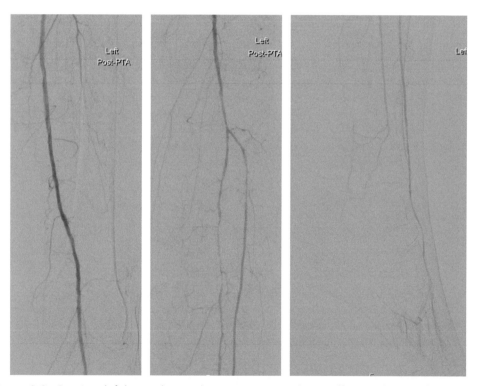

Figure 3.2 Previous left leg endovascular intervention with run-off views down to foot.

The patient has a vascular anaesthetic consultant review. He also has an echocardiogram and pulmonary function tests. The opinion is that this patient is higher than average risk, but if intervention was being considered, a major lower limb amputation would likely be just as risky as a bypass. If surgical intervention was ultimately decided upon, the patient would likely require a HDU bed post-operatively. Please review the fitness test results (Figure 3.4).

Patient scanned supine on a hospital bed. Within this limitation:-

The left CFV, SFV and popliteal veins appear patent, compressible and competent. No DVT seen.

The left LSV is long and straight (measuring 5mm in diameter) from the SFJ to approximately 50mm below the knee where it narrows to 4mm in diameter and bifurcates.

Figure 3.3   Left leg vein map report.

Conclusions

Left Ventricle:
• The LV wall thickness was normal. Not all regions of the LV were visualised clearly, from regions seen imparession is of severely hypokinetic infero-septum, antero-lateral wall and infero-lateral wall. Overall impression is of moderate LVSD. Visually estimated (subjective) LVEF ~40-45%.
• The diastolic filling pattern indicates pseudonormal LV filling pattern, consistent with elevated LA pressure (Grade: 2).

Aortic Valve:
• ? Tissue AVR in situ (details are unknown and nothing was documented on cardiac history on referral). No aortic valve regurgitation. Valve appears well seated with mildly increased FF velocities suggesting mild aortic stenosis.

Tricuspid Valve:
• Intermediate echo probability of pulmonary hypertension.

Urea & Electrolytes

Result	Value	Units	Ref. Range
Sodium	142	mmol/L	133-146
Potassium	4.7	mmol/L	3.5-5.3
Urea	8.6	mmol/L	2.5-7.8
Creatinine	83	umol/L	49-90
eGFR	61	mL/min/1.73m2	
Set Comment:			eGFR may not reflect true GFR, espe detected.OR an AKI calculation has i

Clotting Screen

Result	Value	Units	Ref. Range
Prothrombin time	13	s	9-14
INR (p=poc)	1.1		
APTT (a=anticoag therapy)	43.6	s	23.5-37.5
APTT Ratio (a=anticoag therapy)	1.4		0.8-1.2
Set Comment:			

Full blood Count FBC

Result	Value	Units	Ref. Range
Haemoglobin	97	g/L	115-160
White cell count	12.02	10^9/L	4.00-11.00
Platelets	343	10^9/L	150-400

Spirometry

Substance		Pred LL	Pred	Meas	% Pred	Z-Score	Z-Score
Dose							
FEV 1	L	1.79	2.36	1.59	67.5	-2.18	
FVC	L	2.26	2.98	2.12	71.1	-1.98	
FEV 1 % FVC	%	67.62	79.63	75.17	94.4	-0.65	
PEF	L/min	260	349	247	70.9	-1.88	
MFEF 75/25	L/s	1.13	2.20	1.30	59.1	-1.35	
FEF 50 % MIF 50	%			107.27			
VC MAX	L	2.53	3.22	2.12	65.9	-2.61	

Figure 3.4   Echocardiogram, spirometry, and blood test results.

What would be your provisional plan at this stage accepting the fitness results highlighted above and in conjunction with the anaesthetic opinion?

✓ A   Left femoral-anterior tibial bypass using ipsilateral GSV.
   B   Left femoral-BK popliteal artery bypass with ipsilateral GSV and on-table AT angioplasty.
   C   Left below-knee amputation.
   D   Left above-knee amputation.
   E   Left through-knee amputation.

The patient proceeds with a left femoral-anterior tibial bypass using reversed ipsilateral GSV with a completion angiogram (see Figure 3.5). How do you think this graft has been tunnelled?

   A Anatomically, i.e. superficial to the sartorius muscle, into the below-knee popliteal space, then across the interosseous membrane.

✓ B Anatomically, i.e. deep to the sartorius muscle, into the below-knee popliteal space, then across the interosseous membrane.

   C Non-anatomically, i.e. along the lateral aspect of the thigh and lateral knee.

   D Non-anatomically, i.e. along the anterior aspect of the thigh and anterolateral knee.

   E Sub-dermal, i.e. under the skin along the medial aspect of the thigh down to the below-knee segment, then across the anterior border of the upper tibia, and then deep into the AT wound.

Day 1–4 post-operatively the patient is consistently spiking temperatures up to 39 degrees. His respiratory rate and saturations are largely in an acceptable range, and his chest x-ray is normal. What would you consider to be a reasonable differential diagnosis for his pyrexia within the post-op context?

   A Reperfusion sepsis, hospital-acquired pneumonia, urinary sepsis.

   B Reperfusion sepsis or urinary sepsis.

   C Urinary sepsis, reperfusion sepsis, or viral infection.

   D Hospital-acquired pneumonia, urinary sepsis, reperfusion sepsis, viral infection, or surgical site infection.

✓ E Hospital-acquired pneumonia, urinary sepsis, reperfusion sepsis, viral infection, surgical site infection, or occult intra-abdominal infection.

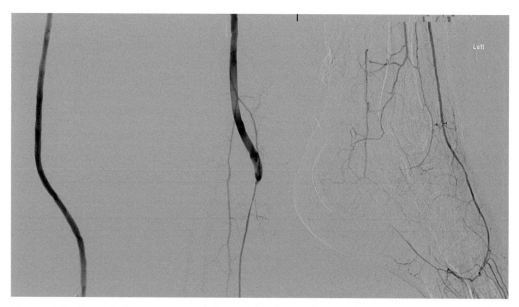

Figure 3.5 Completion angiogram following left femoral-AT bypass using reversed ipsilateral GSV.

The patient makes a timely recovery in the short-term post-operative period with broad-spectrum antibiotics. The working diagnosis was reperfusion sepsis from the left foot which settles with conservative management. He is discharged home around 1-week post-op. Unfortunately, the patient presents 1 month later with deterioration in the left groin wound. There *appears* to be superficial dehiscence of the groin wound. There is a reasonable amount of slough in the wound. There is no clinical infection, the patient's inflammatory markers are otherwise normal, and the patient is systemically well. What is your impression and management plan based upon this information about the left groin wound?

    A This is most likely a full-thickness groin dehiscence (*or at least one that I need to rule out in theatre*). He requires a formal trip to theatre for washout, debridement, and sartorius flap coverage.

    B Superficial groin dehiscence. Oral antibiotics and dressings will suffice.

✓ C Could be superficial or deep dehiscence. I need to do cross-sectional imaging to confirm if there is underlying proximal anastomotic compromise before making definitive surgical decisions.

    D Could be superficial or deep dehiscence. Need to do arterial duplex to confirm if the graft is compromised.

    E Superficial wound dehiscence. Requires a trip to theatre for washout, debridement, possibly for graft ligation +/− above-knee amputation and/or sartorius flap coverage.

What do you make of the CTA imaging of the left groin (Figure 3.6)?

    A Deep fascial layer dehiscence with fluid collection around proximal graft anastomosis.

✓ B Superficial layer dehiscence with no proximal anastomotic compromise.

    C Deep fascial layer dehiscence with proximal anastomotic pseudoaneurysm.

    D Superficial layer dehiscence with gas around femoral vessels indicates necrotising infection.

    E Completely normal CTA.

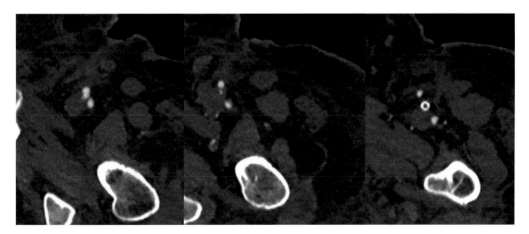

Figure 3.6   CTA of left groin 1-month post-operatively.

The CTA report says that there is a superficial dehiscence but the proximal anastomosis and graft are intact. How would you manage this groin complication?

✓ A Larvae therapy +/– antibiotics.

  B Formal surgical debridement in theatre.

  C Formal surgical debridement and sartorius flap coverage of proximal anastomosis followed by negative pressure wound therapy.

  D Antibiotic treatment alone.

  E Antibiotics and regular dressings.

CASE REFLECTIONS

A relatively young gentleman who is physiologically much older than 56. Multilevel disease bilaterally. He has already lost one leg, and clearly the endovascular attempts for the left leg have not been durable. Extensive medical comorbidity: cardiac, pulmonary, and renal. It does not take a rocket scientist to work out that this patient is in big trouble. However, it was our opinion that he was "fit enough" for a bypass, he did have a viable limb salvage option using decent ipsilateral GSV, and therefore he should be considered for bypass surgery. Ultimately this bypass was successful … although it was not a walk in the park.

The main challenges in this case (*at least from my perspective*) were more in relation to the pre-operative decision-making and the post-operative care, not so much with the operation itself. The pre-operative challenges were mainly in regard to deciding on what was the best revascularisation plan for him. The MRA suggested that he had a long length SFA occlusion, and although the BK popliteal artery appeared to be the natural target for a bypass … the AT origin did appear to be diseased. Indeed, as seen in the prior DSA images, he was known to have had AT origin disease before and this had already been angioplastied. The MRA suggested that this AT origin disease had recurred, and perhaps this "outflow" issue partly explained why his last SFA endovascular attempt had failed (*I am sure the on-going smoking did not help either*). Ignoring the AT for a moment, he also appeared to have peroneal run-off on the MRA, therefore why not consider using this as the main run-off vessel? Or why not consider just bypassing onto the BK popliteal and allowing the run-off to be maintained via the peroneal (*and ignore the AT origin disease*)? The thought process behind the fem-AT bypass was that the AT vessel seemed to be the best vessel running into the foot, the peroneal was occluding at the ankle level, and the notion of doing a BK popliteal bypass and then an additional on-table AT angioplasty just seemed to be making the operation more complicated than it needed to be.

In the end, the fem-AT bypass was otherwise straightforward. The only challenge was the deep groin/slight abdominal apron … but this is not so unusual these days in my experience, and certainly not an insurmountable obstacle. As you can see, there was a very good radiological result. The AT was supplying an almost complete foot arch. The graft was tunnelled anatomically under the sartorius and across the interosseous membrane.

This patient did slightly struggle post-operatively with persistent temperature spikes from day 1 until day 4, along with acute-on-chronic renal impairment and type 1 respiratory failure. However, he improved with appropriate antibiotics and medical support. He never actually required formal intensive care input (*i.e. no intubation or ventilation, no filtration, no inotropic support*). We never found out why he was spiking temperatures immediately post-operatively, but we considered: hospital-acquired pneumonia, urinary sepsis (*related to urinary catheter insertion peri-operatively*), reperfusion sepsis from the left foot, possibly a deep seated surgical site infection, occult abdominal or pelvic sepsis, viral infection … all his cultures were negative, the wounds were all initially fine, and the viral screen was negative. In conclusion I do not know why he was spiking temperatures, but my gut instinct tells me that it was reperfusion sepsis related to the left foot. Although the left foot only ever displayed dry gangrene and no obvious clinical infection, it may well have been the case that he had elusive deeper ischaemic changes in the foot that mounted a systemic inflammatory response immediately post-operatively.

The readmission 1-month post-op with a superficial groin dehiscence was not entirely surprising. However, this was managed with a few days of larvae therapy and things improved without him needing further surgical intervention. There was a deliberate attempt to avoid surgical intervention on this patient because clearly, he was complication prone … and usually if someone is complication prone, this means you should deliberately try to stop poking the bear further!

A challenging case. I think the main reflection points for me relate to the ***recognition of high-risk patients, and ultimately knowing what you are signing up for when you choose to operate on someone.*** Comorbid diabetic patients with cardiac, respiratory, and renal disease (*and a deep groin*) are likely to encounter such post-operative complications after major vascular surgery, so expect it and be prepared for it. I would also emphasise however that just because someone is comorbid, is at high risk, and has already lost one leg, this does not necessarily mean the patient should be deprived of a limb salvage attempt. This patient was about as comorbid as they get, and it was not an easy ride … but he did get off the rollercoaster with his left leg intact. Therefore, at least in this case, palliation and major amputation were not his only options.

A 24-year-old patient presents to A&E with bleeding from the right groin at 7.30 pm. The patient is an intravenous drug user, and also has a background of previous lower limb DVTs. You are told that the patient looks pale and there is a fresh blood clot and some "ooze" overlying a right groin sinus. The patient has been oozing on and off from the groin for the past week. You are informed that they are haemodynamically stable (heart rate 74, blood pressure 110/70 mmHg). The patient is not septic and there is not reported to be any obvious cellulitis or collection or crepitus in the groin. With this brief information provided, what is your primary working diagnosis?

   A Infected ileofemoral DVT with venous fistula to skin.

   B Superficial groin abscess with superficial venous ooze.

   C Femoral artery pseudoaneurysm that has ruptured.

✓ D Femoral artery pseudoaneurysm with herald bleeding.

   E Necrotising fasciitis with erosion of venous tributary in groin.

What would be your immediate management plan?

   A Blood transfusion, consent and book for right groin exploration and CFA repair using a bovine patch first thing tomorrow morning.

   B NBM, bloods (FBC, U&Es, LFTs, clotting, G&S), crossmatch 4 units of blood, permissive hypotension approach currently, consent form 1, incision and drainage of right groin abscess and haemorrhage control, take to theatre within next 30 minutes.

   C Focused history and examination of the patient, consent form, then rush to theatre immediately for a lower midline laparotomy (for proximal control) followed by ligation of femoral vessels.

✓ D Focused clinical assessment, rapid work-up (bloods, crossmatch a few units of blood), urgent CT angiogram, transfuse if patient is profoundly anaemic, with a likely plan to take to theatre for Rutherford Morrison control of right EIA followed by right femoral vessel ligation.

   E Refer patient back to A&E. Refuse to accept this patient or see them until they have had a CTA.

You go see the patient immediately because A&E already performed a CTA and they are referring the patient with the result already available. What do you make of the CTA images (Figure 4.1)?

   A Normal femoral artery but there is a collection of pus anterior to it (suitable for incision and drainage by general surgeons).

✓ B Psoas sign. Haematoma/pus around femoral vessels. Pseudoaneurysm visible.

   C Necrotising infection around femoral vessels but not pseudoaneurysm. Arrows on CTA represent junction of SFA and PFA.

   D Normal femoral vessels but evidence of infected ileofemoral DVT. Arrows on CTA point to a retained needle in the groin around the femoral bifurcation.

   E Massive mycotic CFA aneurysm.

DOI: 10.1201/9781003497042-4

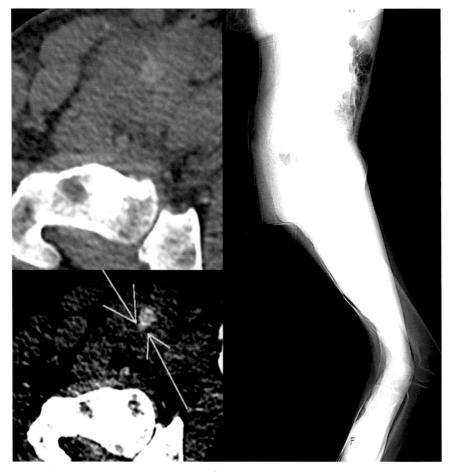

Figure 4.1 CT angiogram and scout x-ray of legs.

You speak to the patient. What are two crucial bits of information you should routinely seek in this specific context?

   A Do you inject in any other sites, and have you had surgery in your groin before?

   B When was the last time you injected, and is there likely to be a retained needle in the groin?

✓ C Are you known to have any bloodborne diseases such as HIV or hepatitis, and are you on any blood thinning medications for previous clots in your legs?

   D Do you smoke, and what is your current social set-up?

   E Do you have any lower limb ulcers, and are you currently on methadone?

The patient informs you that they have previously been treated for hepatitis, and they are now "in the clear." The patient also confirms she has had DVT's in both legs before, and they are usually on a tablet called edoxaban. They say that they last took the edoxaban 2 days ago – and stopped taking it because it did not seem to be a good idea to take a blood thinner while there was active bleeding from their groin (*wise move!*). What would be your management plan now?

✓ A Liaise with haematology in regard to the edoxaban, and update the emergency theatre team that everyone should double-glove and wear eye protection.

B Assume the edoxaban is cleared from their system and do not liaise with haematology. Update the theatre team that the patient is free of bloodborne viruses and nobody needs to take any precautions.

C Delay their operation for a further 24 hours to allow the edoxaban to fully clear from the patient's system. Don't mention to anyone about the previous hepatitis status because it is now all in the clear.

D Avoid operating on this patient because they are at a high risk of carrying other blood-borne viruses and also because they are anticoagulated. A conservative management approach seems more appropriate because they only have a small CFA pseudoaneurysm.

E The edoxaban is very likely to be cleared from the patient's system. However, as they are at a higher risk from a bleeding perspective and a higher risk for bloodborne infections, refer the patient to interventional radiology for a contralateral retrograde femoral approach with a view to covered stenting of the right CFA.

Here is the haematology advice:

Please send urgent edoxaban level to check if it has cleared. If less than 50 most of it has cleared, if higher levels, then please rediscuss. If the patient needs to go to surgery urgently then go ahead without waiting for the results as it will be a matter of risks vs benefits and she has a local cause of bleeding that can be treated. However, if bleeding and going to theatre urgently then please rediscuss urgently as we might have to reverse her edoxaban without having levels available. Can give vitamin K 10 mg IV once a day for 3 days from now. It will take 4–6 hours to work however worth giving and it is not prothrombotic. Tranexamic acid 1g stat unless contraindicated.

With a haemoglobin of 69, otherwise normal renal function, haemodynamic stability but with trickling of blood from the right groin, what would be your management plan?

✓ A In A&E transfuse the patient a few units of blood, give vitamin K 10 mg stat, give tranexamic acid 1 g stat, and then take the patient to theatre as soon as possible (*not waiting for the edoxaban result because pragmatically it has likely been cleared from the system and you cannot afford to wait around forever here as the groin is at high risk of blowing imminently. You can still liaise with haematology however as they may want to reverse the edoxaban without the level available*).

B Take the patient straight to theatre and start operating as the anaesthetist is giving blood, vitamin K, and tranexamic acid.

C Take the patient to theatre immediately, perform the operation to achieve bleeding control, and then transfuse blood and give vitamin K with tranexamic acid afterwards.

D Give the patient a few units of blood, vitamin K, and tranexamic acid, but wait in A&E until the edoxaban level is confirmed. Only then take the patient to theatre once you are 100% confident that the edoxaban levels do not need correcting.

E Give the patient 6 units of blood, vitamin K, tranexamic acid, wait for the edoxaban level to be confirmed, but plan to take the patient to theatre the following day when the patient has been supremely optimised.

You arrive in theatre after the patient has had 2 units of blood (*given STAT in A&E*) and vitamin K, and tranexamic acid. You bring the patient up to theatre yourself. The patient is anaesthetised fairly quickly. More blood is available. The patient is catheterised. They have already had appropriate intravenous antibiotics. How would you plan your surgical approach?

    A Vertical groin incision. Dive straight in – "smash-and-grab" approach.

    B Start with lower midline laparotomy and control right common iliac artery. Then expose SFA and PFA before "attacking the injury." Plan to washout, debride, and repair this false aneurysm using an ipsilateral GSV patch.

✓ C Start with a Rutherford Morrison incision and control the right EIA. Then do an upper thigh incision below the sinus and control the SFA, following that further up to try and control the PFA. Then "attack the injury."

    D Contralateral femoral access, up and over approach, and balloon occlusion of the right EIA. Then vertical right groin incision with "smash-and-grab" approach, i.e. dive straight into the false aneurysm and ligate everything.

    E Lower midline laparotomy, clamp the right EIA, then distal control of SFA and PFA, then "attack the injury" and ligate the distal EIA and proximal CFA. Leave the SFA and PFA origins intact. Then proceed to do a right CIA to SFA/PFA origin prosthetic bypass, bathe it in antibiotic solution, and cover with a sartorius flap.

You do a Rutherford Morrison incision and control the EIA. You make your second incision distal to the groin sinus and expose the SFA underneath the sartorius muscle. You follow the SFA upwards to try and find the PFA, but you encounter what can only be described as a *bloody mess*. There is a load of infected haematoma and necrotic tissue. The tissues are also quite thick and indurated. The tissue planes are grossly abnormal. There is also a lot of venous hypertension and massive venous tributaries that seem to bleed profusely every time you try to dissect further to improve your vision and access. You simply cannot find the PFA. You therefore clamp the EIA and SFA and proceed to "attack the injury." As you excise the groin sinus and dissect deeper into the area of "badness" you suddenly encounter fairly profuse bright red bleeding. The CFA seems to be disintegrated and you assume this impressive bleeding must be coming from the PFA. What would be your plan of attack?

    A Get your assistant with a "swab on a stick" and a big sucker. They press down with the swab and suck as you try to dissect around the area and create some space for you to get a massive Prolene suture (*with a massive needle*) to under-run the CFA/PFA.

    B Just keep sucking away at the bleeding point until the bleeding slows down and you can then see better to suture the PFA/CFA.

    C Get exasperated (*slightly*) and inform your assistant that if they keep sucking away and not using the swab on the stick to compress the bleeding point they are going to exsanguinate the patient.

    D Throw some massive blind Prolene sutures around the area to try and get purchase on the bleeding point.

✓ E *Realistically a combination of A and D (don't admit to C).*

Around 3 minutes later you somehow have stopped the bleeding. What would be your critical next steps?

✓ A Ensure you have achieved haemorrhage control and that all your sutures are secure. Then ensure you have achieved sepsis control, i.e. not leaving behind any abscess cavities deep in the thigh.

B Washout with a few litres of warmed normal saline.

C Sartorius flap coverage of the ligated femoral vessels.

D Making sure you did not cause any small bowel injury at the time of your Rutherford Morrison incision and that the peritoneum is fully repaired (*if you did injure it*).

E Making sure you know what the edoxaban level is.

You are probing with your finger into what appears to be a tract/sinus behind the ligated femoral vessels. There does appear to be a cavity running deep into the thigh. You insert a few fingers and attempt to open it up by being "assertive." Some pus comes out and you therefore insert your hand into this large cavity. You drain some obvious pus and feel like you have definitely done the right thing. You insert your fingers deep inside this cavity and start sweeping left and right to make sure any loculations are broken down. Suddenly, torrential dark red blood starts pouring upwards out of this cavity. What do you think has happened and what are you going to do next?

A Stick the sucker inside and see if you can see the bleeding point to oversew.

B Get a massive pack and stick it deep inside the cavity, and then manually compress thigh from outside using both your hands (*to tamponade the bleeding point*).

C Open the cavity longitudinally (down the thigh), insert a deep self-retainer, and then once you can see the bleeding point oversew it using a massive Prolene suture.

D Don't panic – it is likely to just be a small venous bleed. Just stick a massive pack in and plan for its removal on the ward in 48 hours (*as it will have stopped bleeding by then*).

✓ E Combination of B and C.

You open up the deeper thigh compartment and insert a deep self-retainer (*packing and compression did not stop it bleeding*). There is a large venous structure that has been transected and both ends are hosing blood. The veins themselves look inflamed and thin walled. What would your management plan be here?

A End-to-end anastomosis using 5-0 Prolene (*i.e. repair the injury*).

B Shunt the veins together and plan to bring the patient back for prosthetic interposition graft repair in 24 hours.

✓ C Get another massive Prolene suture and oversew both bleeders.

D Ligate the injured veins using a 3-0 vicryl tie.

E Suture ligate both injured veins using 7-0 Prolene.

CASE REFLECTIONS

A classic emergency vascular surgery case. These cases teach you almost everything you need to know about vascular surgery (*we will run through each theme separately*):

- Pragmatism.
- Importance of history and examination.
- Proximal control, distal control, then attack the injury (*i.e. vascular trauma principles*).
- Sepsis control.
- How to deal with challenging bleeding (*arterial and venous*).
- Different methods of wound closure.
- Classic pitfalls in vascular surgery.

Pragmatism

I will not labour the point here, but ultimately these IVDU groins do explode. If there is an open sinus with blood seeping out you are literally just waiting for it to go bang. You can either ligate the femoral vessels before the fact, or after the fact. If you have a patient with herald bleeds who is a bit anaemic and there are some minor clotting concerns then I think it is reasonable to spend a *bit* of time optimising the patient pre-operatively. In the case above it was a good move to give them some blood and tranexamic acid and vitamin K because they did end up bleeding in theatre. However, the notion of waiting around forever for some edoxaban result or waiting for the following morning when the haemoglobin was 140 just feels a bit risky. From guidelines that our department uses, I already know that with reasonable renal function most of the edoxaban would have been cleared within 2–3 days anyways. The patient was chronically anaemic anyways so I was not aiming for a completely normal haemoglobin pre-operatively. Therefore I made a decision to give the patient a few units of blood, vitamin K, and tranexamic acid, and then just take them to theatre. I would rather take someone to theatre with a *minor* clotting issue than not take someone to theatre until the clotting was perfect, only for the patient to then blow their groin. I think the blood loss and chances of a negative outcome are going to be worse with the latter approach.

*** *This does not mean I am advocating ignoring the influence of anticoagulants. If a patient has as INR of 12 and you rush that patient to theatre for major arterial surgery, I would consider that negligent. Pragmatism is a real-world and balanced approach, it is not a maverick approach.*

Importance of History and Examination

You will be surprised how many IVDUs are on anticoagulants. Many of them have had previous DVTs or PEs. Many will have leg ulcers indicating post-thrombotic syndrome and venous hypertension. You should aim to pick up these clues during your clinical assessment. They are very helpful clues, and the patient in this case quite literally did have leg ulcers, previous DVTs, post-thrombotic syndrome, and was on edoxaban. It was only because the history and examination process picked up these clues that we were aware of the need to consult haematology, and that we should expect venous hypertension and an increased risk of venous bleeding during this operation.

Proximal Control, Distal Control, Then Attack the Injury

For the vast majority of IVDU groin problems my standard approach is to do a Rutherford Morrison exposure to enable me to control the EIA. In some cases you can get control with a vertical groin incision that enables control of the CFA at or just underneath the inguinal ligament. However, in my experience, the IVDU groin almost always is inflamed/indurated, there is often a sinus, and getting the CFA controlled can be tricky. I would rather just get proximal control in clean or virgin territory. The other benefit of routinely using the Rutherford Morrison exposure is that you get slicker at it.

For distal control I would take Sartorius down and just find the SFA underneath it. Then I will track the SFA upwards and try to find the PFA that way. I must however confess from experience that I often cannot find the PFA to sloop it, and I often have to go into the pseudoaneurysm in order to control the backbleeding PFA. This can be tricky, and sometimes the PFA cannot be seen. Exposure of the PFA can also be really tricky. It is hard for me to suggest definitive "hard and fast" solutions for when you attack the injury. My broad advice is to have your assistant with a big sucker, a swab on a stick, and you have a massive Prolene suture in your hand. This is one of the reasons not to blindly rush an IVDU to theatre if they are not actively bleeding ... *as* ***they can still bleed a lot in theatre***. If you start with a decompensated patient, you may end up decompensating them a lot more on table!

Sepsis Control

Watch out for deeper abscess cavities that can track down to the femur/pelvis. Also watch out for abscess cavities that can track along the ileopsoas, underneath the inguinal ligament, and into the retro-extra-peritoneal space. Finally watch out for sepsis that is tracking down the thigh medial and anterior fascial planes towards the knee. Do not be afraid to make bold incisions and make sure the sepsis has been cleared effectively first time around. If you have only made a laparoscopic-sized incision now and have not truly achieved sepsis control, all that means is that your colleagues are likely going to be in at midnight in 48 hours' time extending that incision and releasing a gallon of pus.

How to Deal with Challenging Bleeding

Focusing specifically on this case, it must be emphasised that **the basics must be applied first of all**. It is a total waste of time focusing on the minutiae of haemorrhage control and expecting a successful outcome if the patient is over-anticoagulated and you have not achieved proximal and distal control of the main feeding arteries. These things must come first.

In this case we encountered troublesome PFA back bleeding, along with a pseudo-iatrogenic SFV injury. Both these vascular injuries initially could not be seen, and they were initially inaccessible. This is actually what I believe constitutes truly challenging bleeding – you cannot see it, you cannot access it. Therefore, you need a more pragmatic approach, and here are seven possible options you can try:

1) Apply direct pressure (above/below/from the right/from the left/directly on top).
2) Try packing the area +/− broad manual compression using young hands.
3) Get decent suction to aid your vision.
4) Enlarge your wound and/or dissect around the bleeding point to make it more accessible.
5) Use retractors/self-retainers to aid your vision.
6) Use a massive Prolene suture and to try and grasp the soft tissues that are surrounding the likely source of bleeding in order to bring everything together en masse (*i.e. a tamponade effect*).
7) Sometimes relatively blind deep suturing is all you can realistically achieve – and in the appropriate context it may be the correct course of action (*but don't apply this principle in critical areas such as around the root of the small bowel mesentery*).

Different Methods of IVDU Groin Wound Closure

There are loads of different options for the IVDU groin that you have just performed a triple-vessel ligation on. I will tell you my standard approach:

1) Washout the groin with at least 2 litres of warmed normal saline.
2) Sartorius flap coverage of ligated femoral vessels.
3) Corrugated drain goes underneath the Sartorius bed and is allowed to come out of the mid-section of the wound.
4) 2–0 vicryl continuous to fascia and clips to skin – but leave mid-section of groin wound open.
5) Betadine soaked Caesarean section roll to mid-section of wound and then pressure-dressing on top.
6) NPWT to mid-section of wound at 48 hours.
7) If the infection in the groin has been absolutely catastrophic I will likely just pack the entire wound with Betadine-soaked Caesarean section roll with a view to a re-look in theatre in 48 hours time.

Classic Pitfalls in Vascular Surgery

Here are just a few "theoretical" examples I am aware of:

- Rushing an IVDU to groin because of herald bleeds but patient is not optimised, i.e. already quite anaemic and surgeon did not realise patient was on warfarin. Patient bleeds out on table.
- Trying to get proximal control in groin and struggling, then when blood loss ensued +++ having to convert to Rutherford Morrison incision to get EIA control.
- Not realising there was a retained needle in the groin (*retrospectively visible on CTA*) and poor surgeon getting a needle stick injury.
- Surgeon not wearing eye protection and getting blood in their eye – patient turned out to be HIV positive.
- Oversewing the PFA using a large Prolene suture. Haemostasis achieved according to operation note; 45 minutes later patient is rushed back into theatre because of fairly significant bleeding in theatre recovery. The PFA had only been 50% oversewn. Indeed, a set of forceps probed into the PFA confirming it was still patent. A very quick but more assertive massive Prolene suture solved this problem – but lesson learnt.
- Endovascular management of the IVDU groin pseudoaneurysm, i.e. the covered stent in the CFA. Initially impressive result … until 4 weeks later the patient is back in theatre with a massive infected pseudoaneurysm and an infected free-floating CFA stent. Moral of the story here is do not put prosthetic material in the IVDU groin.
- Prosthetic repair of the IVDU femoral pseudoaneurysm. There will always be someone who supports this approach, but it is not being advocated in this book.
- The IVDU who has the "abscess in the groin" with a CTA that shows it is sitting behind the femoral vessels. The patient is currently under the general surgeons in another hospital and they are asking if vascular are happy to take the patient over. In this instance I have seen cases where vascular surgeons have pushed back and said that general surgery should take the case on or ask interventional radiology to do an ultrasound-guided drainage. I am not so fussed about the IR approach although slightly cynical about its efficacy. However, in regard to the general surgeons operating behind the femoral vessels … nah. If I got a phone call like this I would just take the patient. I am aware of vascular surgeons who have advised the general surgeons to take the patient to theatre and the vascular surgeon will be around to assist if necessary. However, all I will say is that IVDU groins can be tricky and risky, and if there is any concern about possible bleeding (*i.e. iatrogenic vascular injury*) or vascular involvement I have a low threshold to accept these patients under my care.
- Taking a stable IVDU groin patient to theatre without a CTA. I would always recommend a CTA if you have the opportunity. The hosing groin clearly does not apply in this context, but apart from that I think a CTA will quite simply help you. It will tell you if the problem is in the groin, is it extending above the inguinal ligament, if there a deeper collection in the thigh, if there is a retained needle in the groin …? For example, if there was a massive CFA pseudoaneurysm that extended up to the proximal EIA, you may instead choose a lower midline laparotomy to get proximal control of the CIA (*instead of the Rutherford Morrison approach*).

You are the vascular consultant on-call. It is 6 pm. Your phone rings, and there is a panicked voice on the other end. It is a general surgery registrar speaking on behalf of an upper GI surgery consultant who is requesting immediate vascular surgery assistance. The referring team are from an adjacent hospital that you provide vascular surgery cover for (*but this hospital has no routine vascular surgery presence on-site, and there are no regular major elective vascular surgery procedures performed here*). This hospital is around a 10-minute car drive away. The registrar on the phone is speaking very fast, and it is hard to fully make sense of what is going on. You are informed that they are currently in theatre with a 48-year-old female patient who it sounds like has had a complex gastric cancer resection. There is now major bleeding from what they think is a superior mesenteric vein. The patient is haemodynamically unstable. The bleeding site is packed and currently controlled with pressure. The referral is quite confusing, and you are confronted with a load of panicked complex information in a very short period of time. All you can grasp is that *this is a relatively young woman with a gastric cancer that has been resected, the dissection was difficult, there is now fairly impressive venous bleeding in the upper abdomen, and the patient is unstable.*

How are you going to respond to this?

   A Panic yourself and immediately get in the car and speed off in the direction of the referring hospital.

   B Explain to the registrar that you need more information. Ask about pertinent details of the operation, how long has it been going on, who is doing the operation (*name of the consultant*), which theatre they are in, confirm the hospital, confirm how unstable the patient is (i.e. is the lethal triad of hypothermia, coagulopathy, and acidosis present), and what have they done already to try and stop the bleeding?

✓ C Explain to the registrar that you need more information. Ask limited details about the operation so you can orientate yourself (*e.g. was this purely open surgery or laparoscopic*), what is the name of the consultant, which theatre they are in, confirm the hospital, and confirm how unstable the patient is. Instruct the registrar that there is going to be a 10–20-minute delay before you arrive and you need a contact phone number in case you cannot find the theatre/changing room. Write the pertinent details down on a piece of paper in case you forget. Instruct the team to activate the major transfusion protocol, to call for other senior surgical support from any adjacent theatres, to put a finger on any bleeding areas (*or pack and apply general pressure*), and to open up a vascular tray and have some Prolene sutures ready.

   D Seek extensive details about the operation and specific anatomical details about the suspected vascular injury. Instruct the team to activate the major transfusion protocol and to pack the area with loads of swabs until you arrive. Tell them that if they cannot achieve control to simply get some massive Prolene sutures and proceed with some blind enormous stitches to try and oversew the bleeding point. Tell them you will be in theatre in about 15–20 minutes.

   E Confirm which hospital it is, which theatre it is, and what is the name of the operating consultant. Explain that you need a contact phone number in case you cannot find the theatre/changing room. Write this key information down on a piece of paper. Instruct the team put a finger on the bleeding point (if it is visible) or just to pack the area. Advise the team to activate the major transfusion protocol, to call for other senior surgical support from any adjacent theatres, open a major vascular tray, and get some Prolene sutures ready. Tell them you should be there in about 20–25 minutes.

DOI: 10.1201/9781003497042-5

The traffic is relatively busy. As you are approaching the hospital there is a small traffic jam. How would you respond?

A Start honking your horn and revving your engine. Hopefully this will clear the traffic jam.

B Mount the kerb and go around the traffic jam.

C Pull your car over on the side of the street and run to the hospital (*it is around a 5-minute run away*).

✓ D Be patient and stay calm and wait for the traffic jam to clear.

E Roll your window down and start shouting and swearing at the drivers in front of you, screaming that a patient is bleeding to death and you are a consultant vascular surgeon who needs to get out of this traffic jam ASAP.

The traffic jam actually clears fairly quickly and you arrive in the hospital car park 3 minutes later. You quickly walk into the main reception area. There is nobody at main reception to guide you to theatres. You walk towards the main elevator site and quickly peruse the signs to see where theatres are. Bizarrely, the signs/map indicate where every other department in the hospital is, but it genuinely does not say where theatres are (or maybe it does and you just cannot see the sign). You ring the telephone number that was provided for you to call, but there is no phone signal. You look around and cannot see anyone wearing a staff uniform. You ask a random person for help, and they tell you they have no idea where theatres are located. What would you do now?

✓ A Find a member of staff and ask for help with directions.

✓ B Reflect upon how utterly ridiculous it is that some bright spark who designed the sign for the hospital departments decided not to indicate where theatres are located!

✓ C Look confused and disoriented and helpless in the hope that somebody will help you.

✓ D Pray for help.

✓ E Stay calm and accept that you can only do what you can do. If theatres are not signposted clearly how on earth are you supposed to know where they are located?!

A pleasant woman who is passing by sees that you are lost. She is dressed in civilian clothes. She asks if you need help. You explain that there is a patient bleeding to death in theatre and you are a vascular surgeon who has been called to come and help, but you have no idea where theatres are. She then explains that she actually works in theatre and is heading home after her shift, but she will take you to theatres now. She walks you into theatre recovery and hands you over to the recovery nurse there. The recovery nurse informs you that he was aware that there was a vascular problem in theatre, that the operation has been going on for quite a few hours, and that he was aware a vascular surgeon had been called. He walks you around to the changing rooms and lets you in. You change into scrubs and then are escorted into theatre. As you walk into theatre you see quite a few surgeons, a few anaesthetists, and another consultant vascular surgeon who is actually a colleague. What would be your approach?

A Don't talk to anyone. *Actions speak louder than words.* Just scrub in immediately and get to work.

B Introduce yourself to the anaesthetist first. Ask how the patient is doing i.e. is the lethal triad being displayed (acidosis/coagulopathy/hypothermia)? Ask if the major transfusion protocol has been instituted and are they giving blood products in a 1:1:1 ratio? Then introduce yourself to the surgical team and get a brief update. Then go and greet your vascular consultant colleague, devise a mini-strategy together, and finally scrub in and get to work.

C Ignore the anaesthetist(s) and only talk to the surgeons in the room.

✓ D As you walk into theatre "read the room." If things seem relatively calm then decide to introduce yourself to colleagues, seek more information, and plan your attack. If things seem desperate then scrub in very quickly.

     E Walk into theatre and start raising your voice and asserting your authority. Appear stressed and similarly come across as intimidating.

The theatre feels relatively calm. The anaesthetist says the patient is reasonably stable, there is no lethal triad, and they already have blood, fresh frozen plasma, and platelets in the room ready for transfusion. There are three upper GI surgery consultants scrubbed in and a fourth on-call surgical consultant unscrubbed providing moral support. Your vascular surgery consultant colleague is scrubbing in currently. There is a laparotomy wound that is not fully extended. The abdomen is packed. You are told that bleeding is currently controlled. What questions should you ask of the upper GI surgeons?

     A What do they think the vascular injury is?

   ✓ B What operation have they done, where is the injury anatomically located, and what do they think the vascular injury is?

     C How long has the operation been going on for, when did this injury occur, and how have they tried to fix it?

     D Do they think this was an iatrogenic laparoscopic injury or was it at the time of conversion to open surgery?

     E How furious will the bleeding be when the packs are removed?

The upper GI surgeons explain that a laparoscopic partial gastrectomy was planned, but there was bleeding identified during a "difficult dissection." The transverse colon was involved in the malignant process and also required resection. During this long and complex surgery bleeding was encountered in the right upper quadrant that could not be controlled laparoscopically. The surgeons quickly converted to open surgery via a midline laparotomy, but they still could not control the bleeding. The injury is difficult to confirm but there is furious dark venous bleeding in the right upper quadrant (*above the pancreaticduodenal complex they inform you*). They think it is the superior mesenteric vein that has been injured. They say there is no expanding retroperitoneal haematoma. See Figure 5.1 for an anatomical description of the site of the injury.

Based upon the anatomy of this area, and the fact that they think this is mainly a major venous injury, *without even seeing the injury,* what do you think is the most likely vascular injury here?

     A Superior mesenteric vein injury.

     B Superior mesenteric artery injury.

     C Middle colic vein injury.

     D IVC injury.

   ✓ E Portal vein injury.

How would you start off your operation?

   ✓ A Make sure that the scrub nurse has a vascular tray open with some suitably sized vascular sutures, and extend your laparotomy superiorly and inferiorly.

     B Allow the general surgeons to remove the packs, and further supervise them as they reveal the vascular injury to you.

     C Insist that theatre provide you with an Omnitract first, otherwise you are not starting to operate.

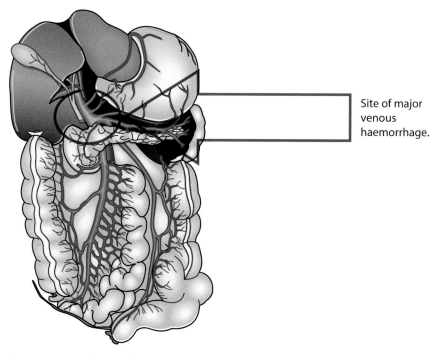

Site of major
venous
haemorrhage.

Figure 5.1   Anatomy of injured area and surrounding structures.

D Grab that knife and swing it upwards. Remove the xiphisternum. Ask the general surgeons to get two big retractors and pull the ribcage upwards. Ask the anaesthetist to insert a nasogastric tube to allow you to feel where the oesophagus is. Then proceed to clamp the supra-coeliac aorta. After this proceed to removing the packs and delineating the vascular injury.

E Get a massive 2-0 Prolene suture in your hand, whip those packs out, and get suturing.

You extend your laparotomy up and down. The vascular tray is already open. There is no Omnitract available but this does not come as a surprise to you as this is a hospital that does not provide routine major arterial surgery. You have loads of assistants however, so retraction is not an issue. You are also advised that there is a second bleeding point that is less severe a few centimetres to the right of the major venous bleeding point. What would you do now?

A Leave the "minor" bleed with the pack applied. Lift the pack off the major bleeding point.

B Leave the major bleed with the pack applied. Lift the pack off the "minor" bleeding point.

C Lift all the packs out at the same time.

D Leave the major bleed with the pack applied. Lift the pack off the "minor" bleeding point for a very short period of time to get an idea of what you are dealing with, then re-apply it and plan your attack.

✓ E Leave the major bleed with the pack applied. Lift the pack off the "minor" bleeding point for a very short period of time and apply finger pressure once you know what you are dealing with.

As you lift away the pack from the "minor" secondary bleed it appears to be a fairly impressive spurter from the transverse mesocolon. There is also venous bleeding coming from the same area. This area is well to the right of the head of the pancreas and duodenum. What would you do now?

  A This is an SMA injury. I need to fully expose this area, get proximal and distal control, and then repair the vessel using great saphenous vein from the groin.

✓ B This is likely a middle colic artery and vein injury. This bad boy is getting oversewn very quickly, and I ain't going to think twice about it. Hand me big vicryl suture please.

  C This is likely to be the right hepatic artery. As the portal vein is possibly injured I am going to have to repair this.

  D This is likely to be the right renal artery. I need convert to do a right nephrectomy.

  E I have no idea what this vessel is. If I ligate it there could be massive ischaemic complications. I am just going to stick a load of clotting products over it and pack it again and hope this stops it bleeding. I am also going to blame the anaesthetist and insist that they speak to haematology and sort out this patient's obvious clotting problem.

After stopping this "minor" spurter from contaminating your field further (*it was a branch of the middle colic artery*), you now have the beast to face. You lift up the pack and indeed there is what can only be described as catastrophic major venous haemorrhage from above the pancreaticduodenal complex. You apply your finger to the bleeding point which appears to be an anterior laceration that is around 6 mm in diameter. There appears to be three large veins converging at this bleeding point. The main vein confluence appears to be intact however (*i.e. this is not a transection*). What should you do now?

  A Ligate this vessel (*i.e. get around it and tie it using a heavy vicryl tie*).

  B Oversew this vessel using a heavy Prolene suture.

✓ C As you apply finger control with one hand and suction the surrounding area with your other hand, enable your vascular surgery colleague to gently clamp the three converging veins.

  D Suction the area while your vascular surgery colleague attempts to repair this laceration using 5-0 Prolene.

  E Suction the area while your vascular surgery colleague attempts to repair this laceration using a 3-0 vicryl suture.

Three gentle vascular clamps are applied to the three converging veins and the bleeding stops. The venous injury is repaired using 6-0 Prolene running suture. The group consensus is that this was a portal vein confluence injury. There is no further bleeding evident. What would you do now?

  A Do a full diagnostic laparotomy and truly confirm there are no further bleeding points. Make sure you rule out a duodenal, pancreatic, aortic, IVC, and hepatic artery injury. If any of the injuries are present (*particularly if you have just caused such injuries by going looking for them in the first place*) make sure they are repaired before you stand down.

✓ B Confirm there is an SMA pulse in the mesentery and then "stand down," leaving the rest of the operation to the general surgeons. Complete a detailed operation note that covers your specific involvement and the context in which you were called to help. Describe in your operation note what specific vascular surgery follow-up/aftercare is required.

  C Go back to the bleeding points after waiting 10 minutes. Aggressively poke and firmly rub the areas of concern just to make sure they are truly secure.

  D Explore the right upper quadrant in detail and insist upon an on-table cholangiogram to make sure there is no common bile duct injury.

  E Instruct the upper GI surgeons to stand down and you will take ownership of the rest of the operation. Explore the abdomen, wash it out, leave drains, close the abdomen etc.

CASE REFLECTIONS

The big points of relevance to take away from this case are thus:

- Make sure you know exactly where you are needed, and who is the consultant surgeon calling you for help. The reason this is critically important is that as you are en route you want to be 100% confident that you are going to the right place. With such pan-icked referrals you may not grasp all the relevant and correct information. It would be a disaster if you misheard the hospital name and went to the wrong place. The relevance of knowing the consultant surgeon's name is that if you misheard which hospital or theatre it was, or forgot which part of the hospital it was, then at the very least you have a *point of reference*. For example, if you misheard the theatre number, when you arrived you could say to the recovery staff or theatre staff: "I have been called to help Mr … or Miss … but I don't know which theatre they are in." Another benefit of knowing the name of the consultant is that if you are lost you can at least telephone the hospital switchboard and ask to be put through to the consultant surgeon's mobile phone, and then hopefully someone in theatre will answer the phone on his or her behalf.
- Know your anatomy. The right upper quadrant is tiger country (*i.e. surgical soul ter-ritory*). You need to know which structures are where, what relation they are to each other, which structures are critical to preserve, and which can be safely ligated. In this case the middle colic vessels can be ligated (*in a damage control setting*), but the portal vein you would rather not ligate. Also, by way of anatomical knowledge, you can already predict what injury this is not likely to be. For example, the superior mesenteric vein runs posterior to the pancreatic head. Therefore, anatomically speaking, such a major venous injury just above the pancreatic head is more likely to be a portal vein injury.
- Use the initial referral as an opportunity to get the upper hand. You can always advise the surgeons to do a laparotomy, press on the bleeding point, apply a pack for a venous injury, give tranexamic acid, open a major vascular tray, get some vascular sutures, call for senior surgical support from adjacent theatres, and active the major transfusion protocol. In this case a consultant vascular surgery colleague was present in theatre prior to your arrival purely because he was assisting with a urology procedure in a the-atre down the corridor, and when you advised the team to "call for other senior surgical support from any adjacent theatres," this resulted in him being alerted. If you had not given any such advice then you may have arrived in theatre to be met with just once consultant general surgeon, no major transfusion packs available, no vascular tray, no vascular sutures, and no senior vascular surgery consultant to assist you. There is no guarantee you will get everything you have asked for … but if you don't ask you almost certainly won't get.
- Have a low threshold to **STAND DOWN** once you have completed your assigned task. Remember that within this context you are a vascular surgeon who has been called to help stop the patient from bleeding to death and/or repair an injured vessel. You are not there to take ownership for the entirety of the operation, you are not there to go looking for further problems (*unless there is a clear indication that there is a further problem that demands your specific attention*), you ideally want to avoid causing further iatrogenic injuries, and you are not needed to repair gastrointestinal injuries if you have gastrointestinal surgeons present. Stick to damage control principles, do your job to the best of your ability, and don't go beyond your mandate would be my advice. Some sur-geons may have a different opinion and that is fair enough. However, with this case as an example, why not go exploring the portal triad to see if there is a common bile duct injury? Why not make sure there isn't a hepatic artery injury? Why not start poking the duodenum and pancreas at the same time to see if there is a perforation or pancreatic

head laceration? Why not do a right medial visceral rotation and start checking that the IVC is intact? Why not do a left visceral medial rotation and check that the aorta is ok? Great idea and you would get points for thoroughness … but this also sounds like a nice recipe to cause damage to probably uninjured structures in the process. **A judgement call ultimately … but always wise to avoid looking for trouble unless you have no choice**.

- The final thing to take from this case is to **NOT RUSH**. You have no control of the roads and the traffic. It may be a dire emergency and a patient may die if you do not arrive in a timely fashion. However, just because this is your perspective on things and it may be the truth (*i.e. this is your first person viewpoint*), this does not mean this is how other people see things (*i.e. the second and third person viewpoints*). If you start honking your horn and getting angry at other drivers you will likely just be seen as a maniac, and/ or get sucked into some violent road rage incident. Similarly, if you "mount the kerb" or speed you are just as likely to run over a pedestrian. I must also emphasise (*from indirect experience*) that even if you do arrive in a timely manner, many of these vascular catastrophes can still result in the patient dying post-operatively from multi-organ failure (*even if you repair the vascular injury successfully*). Also, imagine if you broke the speed limit and accidently ran over a young pregnant woman and killed her and her unborn baby, only to find out that the "vascular catastrophe" was actually a false alarm and you weren't truly needed anyway. In conclusion – **STAY CALM, AND DO NOT SPEED**.

A 60-year-old male arrives in A&E at 9 pm because of repeated episodes of malaena. This A&E department is in a different hospital 20 minutes away. The patient is haemodynamically stable and otherwise well. He is from Europe and is visiting friends who live in the UK. The patient has informed the A&E doctor who is assessing him that he has had multiple vascular surgery procedures on his abdomen and legs. Based upon this very limited information, what do you consider to be the most appropriate differential diagnosis to consider first?

    A Upper GI bleeding secondary to gastritis.
    B Upper GI bleeding secondary to an underlying gastric malignancy.
    C Upper GI bleeding secondary to oesophageal varices.
✓ D Upper GI bleeding secondary to an aorto-enteric fistula.
    E Upper GI bleeding secondary to mesenteric ischaemia.

The A&E team refer the patient to gastroenterology as the patient is well and clinically this does not suggest aorta-bowel fistula (*apparently*). The patient is seen by the gastroenterology registrar who documents this: "*Looks very well for acute aorto-enteric fistula bleed but mindful that it can present with a herald bleed first.*" The gastroenterology registrar arranges for an urgent CT angiogram. The patient has the following scars/signs (*see Figure 6.1*).

What do you surmise is the most likely surgical history for this patient?

✓ A Aorto-bifemoral bypass, nephrectomy on right, external iliac exposure on left (*i.e. Rutherford Morrison incision*), left axillo-femoral bypass, and left AKA.
    B Femoral-femoral crossover, bilateral Rutherford Morrison incisions, left AKA, and laparotomy.
    C Aorto-bifemoral bypass and left AKA.
    D Axillo-bifemoral bypass and left AKA.
    E Aorto-bifemoral bypass, femoral-femoral bypass, and left AKA.

The patient has had a CTA and you are telephoned with the result. What do you make of the images (*Figure 6.2*)? This is the radiology registrar report:

> *There is peri-aortic soft tissue and fat stranding surrounding the thick-walled infra-renal abdominal aorta, possibly corresponding to a mycotic aneurysm. This abuts a loop of small bowel corresponding to the D4 segment of the duodenum. Appearances are highly concerning for an aorto-duodenal fistula. There does not appear to be any obvious contrast extravasation.*

What is your impression now?

    A This is a potential aorto-duodenal fistula. However, the patient is stable and not actively bleeding. He should have an upper GI endoscopy to confirm there is no other cause for upper GI bleeding first.
    B The changes on the CTA are likely just old inflammatory changes related to multiple previous vascular surgery interventions. The patient should remain under the care of gastroenterology and have an upper GI endoscopy.
✓ C The CTA report is alarming and your review of the CTA suggests the possibility of contrast outside of the aorta i.e. these are herald bleeds predicting imminent exsanguination. This is an aorto-duodenal fistula and the patient requires immediate endovascular intervention i.e. a covered aortic stent.

DOI: 10.1201/9781003497042-6

D The CTA report is relatively reassuring in that there is no contrast extravasation. As such the patient should be transferred under vascular surgery for a covered aortic stent the following morning.

E The CTA report is by a registrar and therefore it is not to be taken too seriously. You will wait for the formal consultant report in the morning before you take over this patient's care.

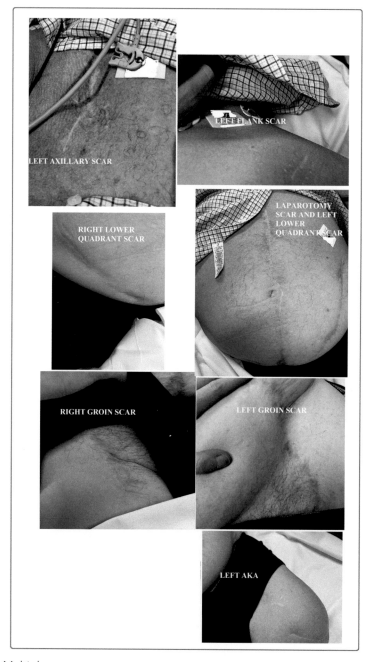

Figure 6.1 Multiple scars.

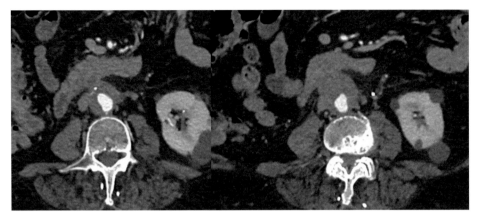

Figure 6.2 Concerning CT angiogram images.

Just for your theoretical interest, here is the formal radiology consultant report from 30 minutes later: "Reviewed and agree with the provisional report. The peri-aortic abnormality abuts the third duodenal segment." What is your plan in terms of patient transfer?

✓ A Accept the patient for ***immediate*** blue light transfer to your hospital. Make patient nil by mouth.

B Accept the patient for transfer to your hospital within the next 24 hours.

C Accept the patient for transfer to your hospital within the next 48 hours.

D Accept the patient for transfer to your hospital within the next 6 hours.

E Accept the patient for transfer to your hospital within the next 12 hours.

You are waiting for the patient to arrive and ask for an update 1 hour later. You are informed that the patient has been assigned as a "category 2 transfer" and that there are significant delays with ambulance services in the region. The patient is still in A&E in the other hospital. How would you respond to this?

A Just be patient. The patient will get here when he gets here. This is not a true vascular surgery emergency as the patient is stable and not actively bleeding.

✓ B Make contact with the clinical site manager of your hospital and highlight that this is a true vascular surgery emergency. The patient may "appear" to be stable but he is having herald bleeds secondary to an aortic mycotic pseudoaneurysm that has fistulated into his small bowel. He is at very high risk of a catastrophic and torrential upper GI bleed any second, and if that happened he would likely exsanguinate and die before intervention could take place. Emphasise that time is of the essence here. Document that you have made these further efforts to expedite this patient's transfer, and also document in very transparent terms that this transfer is an emergency because the patient is at high risk of imminent exsanguination and death.

C Speak to the ambulance service i.e. you ring 999. Try and reason with the 999 operator that this is a very urgent transfer. You are likely to have a very productive conversation.

D You should not have asked for an update on the patient's progress at all. You are just going to rub A&E and the ambulance services up the wrong way.

E Go to A&E in the other hospital yourself and try to move things along that way.

Remarkably after some appropriate escalation the patient turns up around 15 minutes later. You go to see the patient and he is very well, in good spirits, not actively bleeding, and haemodynamically stable. The patient recounts to you that he has had loads of vascular surgery procedures and he shows you all his scars. He also explains that around a year ago he was told he had 5 days to live, he has had an aortic bypass to his groins before, it did get infected, and it sounds like around a year ago he may have had some sort of explantation procedure. He said he has had long-term antibiotics before. He also said that he will try and get access to his previous hospital discharge with all the procedures he has had done. Of note the patient can lie down flat, he only has a right femoral pulse, and he wishes to go ahead with an attempt at covered aortic stent insertion. What would be your current plan of action?

A Try and make complete sense of all the operations he has had done with a very lengthy history and examination.

B Focus on getting the patient out of trouble first with the quickest most expedient method, i.e. covered aortic stent insertion.

✓ C Use your intuition to put the pieces together to vaguely make sense of the situation, review the CTA with vascular radiology, and plan for a covered aortic stent insertion as soon as possible.

D Wait until the following morning, discuss the case in the aortic MDT, and then plan the covered aortic stent when the Portuguese discharge form is available so you know exactly what procedures the patient has had before.

E Palliate the patient because he is clearly at the "end of the line."

You review the CTA with vascular radiology. What do you make of the images (*see Figure 6.3*):

A Occluded left iliac system. Patent and disease-free right ileofemoral system. Patient is suitable for a straightforward right femoral percutaneous covered aortic stent insertion.

B Occluded left iliac system. Patent but diseased right ileofemoral system. Patient is potentially suitable for a right femoral percutaneous covered aortic stent insertion.

C Occluded left iliac system. Patent but diseased right ileofemoral system. Patient is not suitable for a right femoral percutaneous covered aortic stent insertion. Patient requires a re-do right groin exposure, re-do right CFA endarterectomy, bovine patch repair, and then right iliac angioplasty to allow covered aortic stent insertion.

✓ D Occluded left iliac system. Patent but diseased right ileofemoral system. However, it is likely possible for a percutaneous low right CFA puncture and angioplasty of the right EIA to allow covered aortic stent insertion.

E Occluded left iliac system. Diseased right ileofemoral system. This will not allow covered aortic stent insertion from below. Patient requires a re-do left infra-axillary cutdown to allow covered aortic stent insertion from above.

The patient goes for a primary endovascular approach via the right groin. Angioplasty of the proximal CFA and EIA is required to allow covered aortic stent insertion (*see Figure 6.4*).

CASE REFLECTIONS

This case in my opinion is all about "blink" decision-making, pragmatism, and escalation.

"Blink" Decision-Making

Blink decision-making does not require much "over-thinking." It is more about the subconscious application of knowledge, experience, and pattern recognition. In this case the patient

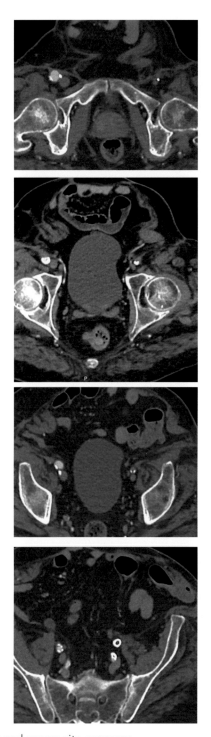

Figure 6.3 CT angiogram and access site concerns.

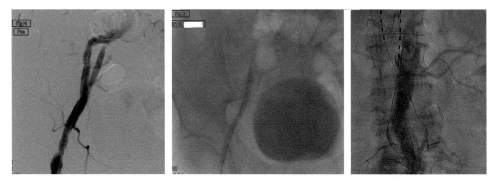

Figure 6.4 Emergency aortic covered stent insertion via right femoral artery.

has had a load of open vascular surgery, he has a midline laparotomy wound, and he is having GI bleeding. Just with these three bits of information one should be able to formulate the diagnosis in around 5 seconds. I do not think you need a hospital discharge form from a foreign country to arrive at the correct conclusion in this context. Indeed, I read the actual hospital discharge form a few days after this patient's admission, and I can barely make any sense out of it (*one because it is in a language I do not speak or read, and two because this patient has had so many complex procedures over the past few years it is hard to make sense of it all anyways*).

Pragmatism
I do not think in this case you really need to know exactly what has been done before. All you need to know are three things:

1) What is the diagnosis (*i.e. aorto-duodenal fistula*)?
2) What is the solution (*i.e. covered aortic stent placement in a timely manner*)?
3) How can I get that covered aortic stent inserted in a timely manner?

The main "pragmatic" things I was interested in when I saw the patient were:

1) Can he lie down flat?
2) Does he have a right femoral pulse with an accessible groin?

The main "pragmatic" things I was interested in from an endovascular perspective were:

1) Is this suitable for a primary percutaneous approach or am I going to have to do a groin cutdown?
2) Can we get away with a less than ideal primary percutaneous approach that avoids the need for a lengthy and difficult re-do re-do re-do groin cutdown and re-do re-do re-do CFA endarterectomy and re-do patch repair?

Escalation
Doors will automatically fly open for patients who are bleeding to death and in grade 4 haemorrhagic shock. However, patients who are literally moments away from being in grade 4 haemorrhagic shock and bleeding to death may not be recognised within the same high priority context (*especially if they are deemed to currently be "stable"*). However, surely it is better to pre-emptively strike and prioritise the patient **NOW** and hit the panic button **NOW**, as opposed to waiting until they become so unstable that their case suddenly becomes an immediate priority (*probably when the horse has already bolted*).

It is important to be aware of this phenomenon, and I would strongly assert that patients within the context of "symptomatic aneurysms" or "herald bleeds" should fit within this truly urgent category. My advice would be to make a fuss out of these patients and escalate the case if you do not feel the patient is getting the proper attention that they deserve. Other clinicians or bed managers or clinical site managers may not understand how urgent the transfer really is (*the classic question would be "How urgent is urgent?"*). Irrespective of different perceptions of how urgent the transfer is, if the patient suddenly ruptures their aneurysm or has a massive upper GI bleed and dies, you may then be exposed to these sorts of questions:

- Why didn't you escalate the patient earlier?
- Why didn't you highlight that the patient was such a high priority?
- Why didn't you say that this was a time critical transfer?
- Why didn't you inform people that these herald bleeds were predicting an imminent catastrophic life-threatening bleed?
- Why didn't you follow up with the patient and ensure the transfer was being prioritised?
- Why didn't you say you were planning an immediate procedure?
- Why did you assume everyone understood how urgent the transfer was?

CASE 7: ACUTE LOWER LIMB ISCHAEMIA

A 42-year-old male presents at 2 am to A&E with an acutely ischaemic right leg. He has reduced power and sensation in his right foot and a tender anterolateral shin compartment. He has a regular and strong ipsilateral femoral pulse but nil distally. His upper limb pulses are normal and regular. His background is that of a previous left leg DVT in 2013 that was deemed to have been provoked (*it was post-op following an inguinal hernia repair*). He did have warfarin after that for a few months, but he is no longer on any anticoagulation. There is otherwise no significant past medical history. He is independent, lives at home with his wife, is a non-smoker, and works as an office manager. There is no relevant family history.

What is your (*most likely*) number 1 differential diagnosis for his acute limb ischaemia?

   A Thrombosed popliteal artery aneurysm.

✓ B Embolic event secondary to cardio-embolic source (*possibly paroxysmal atrial fibrillation*).

   C Type B aortic dissection and subsequent ileofemoral malperfusion.

   D Acute-on-chronic lower limb ischaemia.

   E Embolic trashing from an abdominal or thoracic aortic aneurysm.

The senior A&E physician who first saw the patient suspects the patient has a thrombosed popliteal artery aneurysm. He updated you over the phone initially and explained that he believed the limb was profoundly ischaemic and he needed to go to theatre as soon as possible. He asks you if you think any further imaging is required first. What would you say to the A&E doctor?

   A Further imaging is not going to change management here. The patient just needs to go straight to theatre for a popliteal aneurysm repair or femoral embolectomy.

   B An urgent arterial duplex is required.

✓ C An urgent CT angiogram of the whole aorta and lower limbs is required.

   D An urgent MR angiogram of the whole aorta and lower limbs is required.

   E The patient should go immediately to theatre and you will do an on-table angiogram.

What is your interpretation of the CT angiogram images (see Figure 7.1)?

   A Thrombosed popliteal artery aneurysm.

   B SFA dissection.

✓ C Thrombosed persistent sciatic artery aneurysm with poorly developed SFA and single-vessel PT run-off.

   D Embolic occlusion of distal SFA and compromised run-off.

   E Patent SFA but embolic trashing of crural run-off, with single-vessel PT run-off.

Based upon this formal CTA report (Figure 7.2), what would be your revascularisation plan?

   A Thrombolysis.

   B Prone position and repair of thrombosed persistent sciatic artery aneurysm using inter-position graft, followed by distal embolectomy and calf fasciotomies.

   C Supine position. Below-knee popliteal artery cutdown and embolectomy of thrombosed persistent sciatic artery aneurysm followed by calf fasciotomies.

✓ D Supine position. Right CFA-PT bypass using autologous vein or prosthetic bypass using vein cuff, followed by calf fasciotomies.

   E Intravenous heparin for 24–48 hours. If that does not work, list for primary below-knee amputation.

47

DOI: 10.1201/9781003497042-7

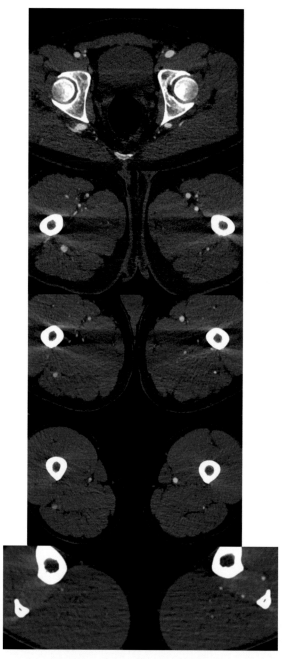

Figure 7.1   CT angiogram for Rutherford 2B right acute lower limb ischaemia.

The patient is taken to theatre and his ipsilateral GSV is of decent quality to be used as a bypass conduit. His popliteal trifurcation is exposed. There is clot in the below-knee popliteal artery. The backbleeding from the PT is only sluggish. What is your surgical approach within this context?

   A Femoral-PT bypass using the ipsilateral GSV.

   B BK popliteal embolectomy and PT embolectomy, femoral-PT bypass using the ipsilateral GSV.

Acute limb ischaemia right lower limb Rutherford 2b, probably thrombosed popliteal aneurysm - for urgent surgery

CT angiogram lower limbs. No prior relevant imaging for comparison.

Normal calibre abdominal aorta with no significant disease. Ectatic but patent iliac vessels. Persistent sciatic arteries bilaterally.

RIGHT:
The persistent sciatic artery can be traced distally to form the popliteal artery (whereas is the right SFA becomes thready and gives off minor collateral vessels in the medial thigh).

As the persistent sciatic artery enters the gluteal region, there is occlusive thrombus along a long segment of approximately 10cm. There is distal reconstitution of flow but with intermittent short segments of nonocclusive thrombus. Short segment of occlusive thrombus at the distal popliteal artery. No flow demonstrated in the anterior tibial artery. Flow within the tibioperoneal trunk, peroneal and posterior tibial arteries to the ankle.

LEFT:
The persistent sciatic artery passes into the posterior thigh and becomes thready with no major branches. The left SFA supplies the popliteal artery. No significant disease in the left lower limb.

Conclusion: Long segment of occlusive thrombus in a right-sided persistent sciatic artery. Images reviewed with Mr   just after scanning.

Figure 7.2   Radiology registrar report of CT angiogram.

C BK popliteal embolectomy and PT embolectomy, femoral-PT bypass using the ipsilateral GSV, and 4-compartment fasciotomies.

✓ D BK popliteal embolectomy and PT embolectomy, femoral-PT bypass using the ipsilateral GSV, ligation of tibioperoneal trunk above the distal anastomosis, and 4-compartment fasciotomies.

E PT embolectomy, femoral-PT bypass using the ipsilateral GSV, and 4-compartment fasciotomies.

What would be your post-operative plan (*please also take into account the CTA addendum report – Figure 7.3*)?

A Closure of fasciotomy wounds and continue single antiplatelet lifelong with routine graft surveillance.

B Closure of fasciotomy wounds, consult haematology for advice in regard to on-going antiplatelet/anticoagulation advice, routine graft surveillance.

C Leave fasciotomy wounds open to heal by secondary intention, no antiplatelet or anticoagulation post-operatively, routine graft surveillance, and bubble echocardiogram.

D Routine graft surveillance and closure of fasciotomy wounds with VOYAGER regime post-operatively (aspirin 75 mg OD and rivaroxaban 2.5 mg BD).

✓ E Routine graft surveillance, closure of fasciotomy wounds, consult haematology for advice on antiplatelet/anticoagulant choice, routine graft surveillance, and discuss contralateral persistent sciatic artery aneurysm in vascular MDT.

Addendum

Review of imaging:

Additional findings:
1. There is evidence of an aneurysm at the site of the thrombosed persistent sciatic artery on the right.
2. There is anomalous venous drainage on the right, with a large venous trunk continuing from the popliteal artery and then along the posterior compartment of the thigh. It eventually joins the deep femoral vein in the proximal thigh.
3. There are varicosites on the left in the similar distribution to the abberent venous trunk seen on the right. I note the patient has had DVT in the left leg 10 years ago. It is possible there was an abberent venous trunk on the left previously which has then been replaced by a collateral network following thrombosis.

Figure 7.3 Consultant vascular radiologist addendum to the CT angiogram.

CASE REFLECTIONS

When I was preparing for my FRCS Part B examination, one of my trainers grilled me with some rare cases, one of which was a young female patient who presented with a Rutherford 2B acutely ischaemic leg. He showed me a weird angiogram which at the time I could not make sense of. The case was actually that of a thrombosed persistent sciatic artery aneurysm in a patient with a patent ileofemoral system but an underdeveloped SFA. This patient had a patent below-knee popliteal artery that was being fed by the persistent sciatic artery. In that case, my trainer basically explained that all he did was a femoral-BK popliteal artery bypass using reversed ipsilateral GSV (*i.e. relatively simple solution for a complex and unusual problem*) …

When our patient here presented to me in the early hours of the morning, I was reviewing the CTA with the radiology registrar on-call, and my initial expectation was that I was going to see a thrombosed popliteal artery aneurysm or a simple embolic occlusion of the SFA. However, there was definitely no popliteal aneurysm, and there was clearly something weird going on … I immediately recalled the case I described to you above of the woman with the thrombosed persistent sciatic artery aneurysm. Call it pattern recognition, but I immediately acknowledged to myself that the patient had a decent femoral pulse, so to get him out of trouble I just needed a decent distal target for a bypass. I telephoned the vascular interventional radiology consultant on-call to check I was OK to bypass onto the PT and confirm that it was a thrombosed persistent sciatic artery aneurysm, and then around 50 minutes later the patient was in theatre with me exposing the groin and the night vascular registrar on-call (*good job Gary*) exposing the TPT …

In this real-life case we did an upstream trawl of the BK popliteal and a load of fresh thrombus came out, to reveal pretty impressive inflow from the path of the persistent sciatic artery. The backflow from the PT was a bit sluggish so to be on the safe side we also trawled the PT and a chunk of fresh clot came out, with the PT backbleeding becoming excellent. We then did a standard fem-PT bypass using reversed ipsilateral GSV with calf fasciotomies. We ligated his tibioperoneal trunk above the distal anastomosis to prevent competitive flow, and also to prevent future embolic events from the persistent sciatic artery down his calf vessels. The patient's fasciotomy wounds were closed 3 days later and he made an otherwise fantastic recovery. His graft is still running over a year later.

We did speak to haematology because he had now had both a venous thrombotic event (*left leg DVT*) and an arterial thrombotic event. The haematology team recommended lifelong DOAC therapy (*direct oral anticoagulation*). We also discussed his contralateral persistent sciatic artery aneurysm in our vascular MDT, and the consensus was that no intervention was required as the contralateral sciatic artery did not connect to the femoral-popliteal system but instead, it mainly peters out into tiny muscular branches (*and thrombosis would likely not lead to significant clinical consequences*).

As a further interesting point in regard to this case, it was felt that his underlying persistent sciatic aneurysms were also a reflection of aberrant lower limb venous anatomy that had likely predisposed him to his left leg DVT. A rare and interesting case.

Final Comment

Now that you have learnt about this case, remember it for your future career. If you come across a relatively young patient with an acutely ischaemic limb and a weird CTA, remember the possibility of a thrombosed persistent sciatic artery aneurysm. If you have a femoral pulse, just look for a decent bypass target … and if you have one, get cracking with a femoral-popliteal/distal bypass!

Figure 7.4 depicts some interesting images showing the thrombosed right persistent sciatic aneurysm, the underdeveloped right SFA, and then the subsequent right fem-PT bypass using reversed ipsilateral GSV.

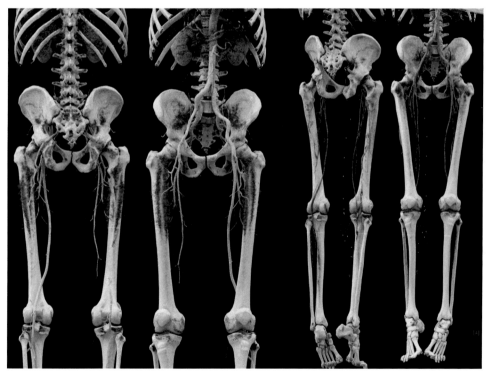

Figure 7.4 3D reconstructions of lower limb CT angiograms before and after right fem-PT bypass using reversed ipsilateral GSV.

A 67-year-old female presents with right foot rest pain and short distance claudication. She is now only able to walk around 40 metres before she has crippling right calf pain. This happened suddenly around 3 days ago. Prior to this sudden deterioration she said she was able to walk around 300 metres before she experienced right calf pain on walking. She is a smoker, hypertensive, has mild/moderate chronic obstructive pulmonary disease (COPD) and hypothyroidism. Her current medications include clopidogrel, levothyroxine, and amlodipine. She lives at home with her husband and is otherwise independent. She is able to move and feel her right foot. She has a soft and non-tender right calf and shin. She has no right leg pulses, with weak monophasic ankle signals. She has no tissue loss. You also cannot feel any left leg pulses but she is otherwise asymptomatic in the left leg. She has normal and regular upper limb pulses.

What is your most likely diagnosis here?

    A Acute embolic right leg ischaemia.

    B Thrombosed right popliteal artery aneurysm.

✓ C Acute in situ thrombosis right leg.

    D Right leg trashing from aortic or thoracic aneurysm.

    E Thrombosed right persistent sciatic artery aneurysm.

What is your immediate management plan?

    A Switch to COMPASS regime (aspirin 75 mg OD and rivaroxaban 2.5 mg BD), advise regular exercise and smoking cessation, and discharge with a plan for outpatient follow-up in 6 weeks.

    B Discharge home on therapeutic low molecular weight heparin with a plan for urgent outpatient CT angiogram lower limbs and urgent outpatient follow-up in 2 weeks.

    C Admit under vascular surgery, full set of bloods, CT angiogram aorta (including arch of aorta) and lower limbs, lower limb vein mapping, analgesia, prophylactic enoxaparin, 12-lead ECG, keep patient nil by mouth, and plan for urgent revascularisation within 12 hours.

✓ D Admit under vascular surgery, analgesia, IV fluids, oxygen, therapeutic enoxaparin, stop clopidogrel and commence aspirin 75 mg OD instead, commence high-dose statin therapy, 12-lead ECG, patient can eat and drink, full set of bloods (*including HBA1c and lipid screen*), CT angiogram aorta (*including arch of aorta*) and lower limbs, lower limb vein mapping, echocardiogram, and pulmonary function tests.

    E Admit under vascular surgery, analgesia, IV fluids, oxygen, therapeutic enoxaparin, stop clopidogrel and commence aspirin 75 mg OD instead, 12-lead ECG, patient can eat and drink, full set of bloods (including HBA1c and lipid screen), MR angiogram lower limbs, lower limb vein mapping, echocardiogram and pulmonary function tests.

DOI: 10.1201/9781003497042-8

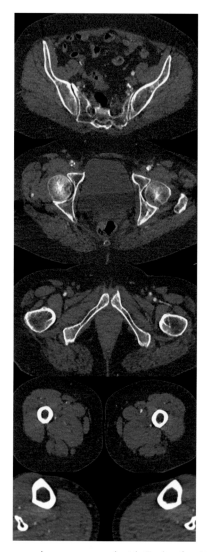

Figure 8.1 Initial CT angiogram when presented with Rutherford 1 ischaemia.

What is your interpretation of the CTA images (see Figure 8.1)?

  A Occluded right iliac system, occluded CFA, patent PFA, long SFA occlusion, 2-vessel run-off via PT and peroneal.

✓ B Occluded right iliac system, diseased but patent CFA, patent PFA, long SFA occlusion, 2-vessel run-off via AT and peroneal.

  C Stenosed right iliac system, occluded CFA, patent PFA, long SFA occlusion, 2-vessel run-off via PT and peroneal.

  D Stenosed right iliac system, occluded CFA, patent PFA, long SFA occlusion, 2-vessel run-off via AT and peroneal.

  E Stenosed right iliac system, occluded CFA, patent PFA, long SFA occlusion, single-vessel via peroneal.

What is your working diagnosis at this junction?

  A Embolic occlusion of the right EIA and SFA.

  B In situ thrombosis of right SFA and right EIA.

✓ C In situ thrombosis of right EIA and chronic right SFA occlusion.

  D In situ thrombosis of right SFA and chronic right EIA occlusion.

  E In situ thrombosis of right EIA and distal embolic trashing of right SFA.

What would be your management plan for this patient currently (*with no tissue loss*)?

  A Conservative management alone with best medical therapy and exercise.

  B Right CFA cutdown, over-the-wire right iliac thrombectomy with right CFA to BK popliteal artery bypass.

✓ C Right CFA cutdown, over-the-wire right iliac thrombectomy +/– iliac stenting, +/– right CFA endarterectomy and profundaplasty.

  D Right CFA cutdown, over-the-wire right iliac thrombctomy +/– iliac stenting +/– right CFA endarterectomy and profundaplasty, +/– downstream SFA over-the-wire thrombectomy +/– SFA stenting.

  E Right percutaneous retrograde iliac stenting alone.

The patient elects for conservative management because she is intimidated by the notion of surgery. She re-presents 4 weeks later with right foot rest pain, night pain, and superficial ulceration over the right 5th metatarsal head with soft tissue infection. She has an unrecordable to pressure with a WIfI stage of 4. In light of her previous CTA, vein map, echocardiogram and spirometry, what would be your provisional/theoretical management plan within this context (*see Figures 8.2 and 8.3*)?

  A Right below-knee amputation.

  B Right above-knee amputation.

  C Right CFA endarterectomy, profundaplasty and iliac stenting.

✓ D Right CFA endarterectomy, profundaplasty, iliac stenting, and likely fem-distal bypass using prosthetic graft and a vein cuff.

  E Right iliac stenting followed by SFA recannalisation (i.e. primary endovascular approach).

Before you commit to your plan, you request a repeat MRA. What do you make of the image and its report (Figures 8.4 and 8.5)? How would you plan your revascularisation approach?

  A Right iliac stent as a staged procedure with DSA of run-off vessels first.

✓ B Right CFA endarterectomy and profundaplasty, bovine patch repair, retrograde EIA stenting, followed by femoral-BK popliteal/TPT bypass using prosthetic graft and a vein cuff with completion angiogram.

  C Right CFA endarterectomy, profundaplasty and SFA origin endarterectomy with bovine patch repair, retrograde right EIA stenting, then antegrade SFA/popliteal recannalisation (+/– stenting).

  D Right CFA endarterectomy, profundaplasty, bovine patch repair, retrograde right EIA stenting, followed by right below-knee amputation.

  E Right percutaneous EIA stenting followed by right above-knee amputation.

The patient had a ***right CFA endarterectomy, profundaplasty, CFA bovine patch repair, right EIA stenting, femoral-peroneal bypass using 6 mm externally supported PTFE graft with ipsilateral GSV Miller cuff and completion angiogram***. Figure 8.6 shows the completion angiographic images.

Spirometry

		Pred LL	Pred	Meas	% Pred	Z-Score	Z-Score
Substance							
Dose							
FEV 1	L	1.53	2.12	1.89	89.0	-0.66	
FVC	L	1.98	2.75	3.11	113.1	0.75	
FEV 1 % FVC	%	64.23	77.85	60.68	77.9	-2.03	
PEF	L/min	250	338	265	78.4	-1.36	
MFEF 75/25	L/s	0.80	1.77	1.07	60.3	-1.11	
FEF 50 % MIF 50	%			32.69			
VC MAX	L	2.24	2.87	3.11	108.1	0.60	

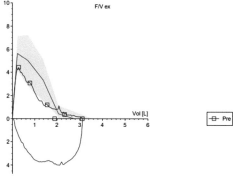

LV size: Unable to accurately measure; visually normal size.
LV function (LVEF/RWMA): Normal/hyperdynamic LV function with visual EF 60-65%. Unable to completely rule out discrete RWMA's.
RV size and function: Where visualised in subcostal window. Impression of good RV Systolic function. TAPSE ranging from 21-24mm.
Valves: Minimally thickened mitral valve leaflet, trivial MR.
TV opens well, Mild TR however from subcostal window moderate TR cannot be excluded.
AV not clearly visualised however normal velocities.

Figure 8.2   Echocardiogram and spirometry results.

Right venous upper limb doppler

The cephalic vein is of poor calibre throughout.

Right venous lower limb mapping

Both the LSV and SSV are of poor calibre.

Left venous upper limb doppler

The cephalic vein is of poor calibre throughout

Left venous lower limb mapping

Both the LSV and SSV are of poor calibre

COMMENTS:
No suitable vein conduit demonstrated within upper and lower limbs.

Figure 8.3   Vein mapping results.

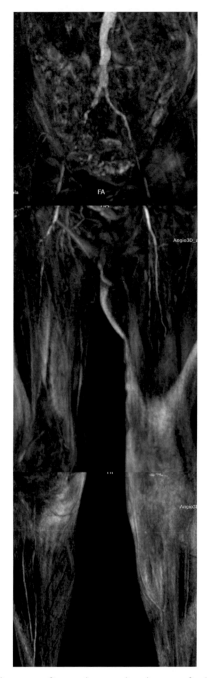

Figure 8.4 MRA lower limbs to confirm a decent distal target for bypass surgery.

Clinical Report
Clinical indication

Right CLTI with tissue loss and infection. No ipsilateral leg pulses. Previous CTA few months ago for right leg Rutherford 1 ALI showed iliac and SFA occlusion, but managed conservatively at that time (working diagnosis was that this was acute iliac occlusion and chronic SFA occlusion). Foot has worsened. She is being admitted for IV abx and work-up for revasc. She has no UL or LL vein for bypass. I suspect she is heading for right iliac stenting and fem-BK pop / distal bypass using PTFE with Miller cuff. Urgent MRA to mainly assess run-off target vessels please.

Report Body

Needs R iliac angio stent   followed by or in same sitting Fem to below knee pop or TP trunk bypass. Peroneal run off with a AT thats diseased and occluded in distal calf. Could do only iliac as PFA run off and see.

Figure 8.5   MRA lower limbs consultant vascular radiologist report.

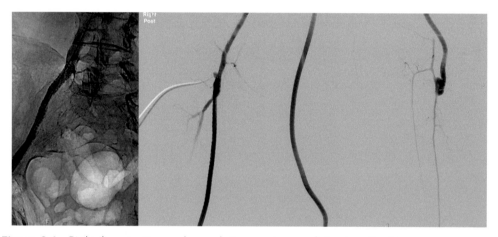

Figure 8.6   Right iliac stenting and completion angiogram following distal bypass.

CASE REFLECTIONS

This patient originally presented with an acutely ischaemic right leg with rest pain and short distance claudication. This was preceded by a fairly classic history of life-limiting right calf claudication at around 300 yards. She had a viable right leg with intact power and sensation and no tissue loss, and she was labelled as Rutherford 1.

Her CT angiogram was slightly challenging to interpret, and there were different postulations at the time. Some thought it might be in situ thrombosis of her SFA with a chronic iliac occlusion, others thought it was in situ thrombosis of her iliac system with a chronic SFA occlusion, others thought it might be in situ thrombosis of her iliac and subsequent distal embolisation down her SFA. The final working diagnosis was that we did not really know, but it was most likely that she had acutely thrombosed her iliac, and the SFA occlusion was likely chronic. Indeed, the notion of a patient occluding both her iliac and SFA and remaining as a Rutherford 1 seemed unlikely (*surely an acute 2-level occlusion would lead to Rutherford 2A or 2B ischaemia*). The revascularisation option presented to the patient was a groin cutdown +/− CFA endarterectomy, and over-the-wire trawl of her iliac system +/− angioplasty stenting. There was an idea to also consider an attempt at over-the-wire trawl of her SFA (*i.e. see if this might be fresh thrombus*) … but in the end the feeling was that as she only had rest pain and no tissue loss then perhaps just clearing her inflow should suffice and get her out of trouble.

However, the patient was somewhat averse to the idea of surgery, and she wanted to manage things conservatively. She was warned that there was a risk of her spending the rest of her life with short-distance claudication, and that she may progress to CLTI. It was also mentioned that in 6 weeks' time we might consider iliac stenting (*once the suspected "fresh" thrombus was no longer fresh*). The patient was subsequently discharged home.

Surprise surprise she presented a few weeks later with full-blown CLTI with tissue loss and infection, sleeping with her leg out of bed, and a Buerger's positive foot. This outcome was predictable, and the patient and her husband were in no doubt now that conservative management had failed and that her options were either major amputation with inflow correction, palliation, or a bypass. We knew she did not have suitable vein and therefore she was going to require a prosthetic bypass. It was made clear to the patient that prosthetic bypasses below the knee are not as durable as vein, and there is an increased infection risk … but there was seemingly no better endovascular option. She was caught between a rock and a hard place, as they say.

In the end she had a positive outcome (*i.e. she kept her leg*). The graft also did not get infected.

Core Considerations/Advice

- Be wary of managing Rutherford 1 acute limb ischaemia conservatively if there is a ***very high chance of a patient progressing to CLTI with tissue loss and if the definitive revascularisation to achieve in-line flow to the foot is going to be very challenging and risky.*** In this case the patient had 4-level disease: iliac occlusion, CFA disease, long SFA occlusion, and crural vessel disease. If her Rutherford 1 acute ischaemia had been treated when she first presented she would likely have just returned to baseline by way of a relatively simple inflow procedure. However, as soon as she progressed to CLTI with tissue loss she was then automatically shunted into needing a complex distal bypass with hybrid involvement and the requirement for a prosthetic graft (*i.e. to achieve in-line flow to the foot*). Do not take this to mean I am suggesting all Rutherford 1 acute ischaemic limbs require intervention – I am categorically not saying this. I am simply saying, maintain a degree of foresight and try to predict what is likely to be the outcome if you do manage things conservatively (***and will the decision to manage things conservatively likely come back to haunt you in a few weeks time?***).
- If you are going to do a distal bypass using prosthetic material be ***meticulous about infection control.***
- Remember that "patient choice" needs to be informed choice. In this case I was quite transparent with the patient in saying that managing her acute limb ischaemia conservatively was potentially a risky strategy, it could come back to haunt her, and I was prepared to offer an inflow correction procedure at the time of the initial presentation. Therefore, the decision-making around the initial conservative management approach was not an "incorrect decision." It was an informed decision by the patient – and there is nothing wrong with that.

A 77-year-old male is referred to you urgently by the general surgery registrar from another hospital. You are told that he has presented with abdominal pain, diarrhoea and vomiting, with a metabolic acidosis and raised lactate. He has diffuse abdominal tenderness but no actual guarding or peritonism. He also has atrial fibrillation on his ECG. What is your working diagnosis?

- A Bowel perforation.
- B Acute appendicitis.
- C Acute pancreatitis.
- D Acute mesenteric ischaemia (thrombotic).
- ✓ E Acute mesenteric ischaemia (embolic).

What further information would you like to know from the referrer (*who is on the other end of the telephone*)?

- A Is the patient stable or unstable? How long have their symptoms been for? What is the past medical history? Have they undergone any cross-sectional imaging?
- B Has the patient had previous abdominal surgery?
- C What is the patient's amylase?
- D What is the troponin and ECG?
- ✓ E All of the above.

You are informed by the general surgery registrar that his symptoms came on around a day ago. He is a good open surgical candidate. His past medical history includes: chronic kidney disease stage 3, iron deficiency anaemia, sciatica, hypertension, type 2 diabetes mellitus, sciatica, myocardial infarction 12 years ago, open appendicectomy, open AAA repair in 2010 (*with a transverse abdominal scar*). The patient lives with his wife, is independent, is an ex-smoker, drinks occasional alcohol, exercise tolerance is around 10 metres due to back pain (*i.e. sciatica*) rather than due to shortness of breath.

What do you make of this CTA (see Figure 9.1)?

- ✓ A Likely embolic occlusion of the proximal SMA.
- B Likely in situ thrombosis of proximal SMA.
- C Mycotic pseudoaneurysm of proximal aortic graft anastomosis.
- D Acute SMA dissection.
- E Acute appendicitis (*please tell me you are joking*).

What are your options at this stage?

- A Keep in parent hospital and advise laparotomy and bowel resection alone (*as there are no options for mesenteric revascularisation*).
- ✓ B Transfer to your vascular unit with a view to either SMA embolectomy or endovascular SMA suction thrombectomy then laparotomy and proceed.
- C Keep the patient in the parent hospital, advise a laparotomy and bowel resection, and you will come across to do an SMA embolectomy.
- D Transfer to your unit for thrombolysis.
- E End-of-life care.

DOI: 10.1201/9781003497042-9

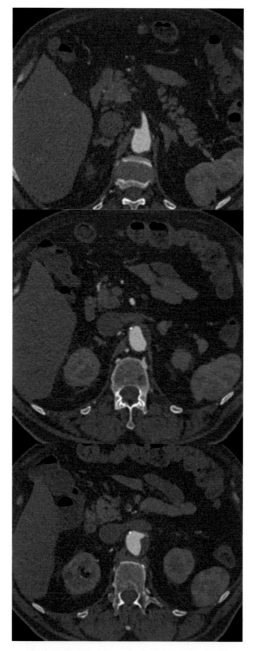

Figure 9.1 CT angiogram of abdomen.

You discuss the case with vascular interventional radiology. The conclusion is that this looks embolic. The patient has threatened gut and needs a laparotomy. Therefore the consensus opinion is that this patient needs an urgent laparotomy and attempt at SMA embolectomy/thrombectomy. You advise for the patient to be transferred over to your hospital immediately (i.e. blue light). When the patient arrives 25 minutes later, he looks clinically well. He has a tender epigastrium, but his pain is out of proportion to the clinical findings, i.e. he is tender ++ but his abdomen is soft and there is definitely no peritonitis. The patient (*and accompanying family members*) agree with the plan to proceed with an attempt at SMA embolectomy.

Where do you think this patient should go to post-operatively?

A Normal ward bed.

B High observation bed (HOBS).

C High dependency unit (HDU).

D Intensive care unit (ICU).

✓ E See how the patient is doing post-operatively, but plan for either HDU or ICU.

What would be your surgical access approach?

A Diagnostic laparoscopy. If bowel looks OK, that is enough. If bowel looks compromised, convert to laparotomy.

✓ B Midline laparotomy.

C Laparotomy through the old horizontal scar (from previous AAA repair).

D Extra-peritoneal approach.

E Left paramedian incision to avoid appendicectomy scar.

What is your provisional plan for revascularisation/bowel resection?

A Bowel resection first, then revascularise, then bowel anastomosis, then close abdomen.

✓ B Revascularisation first, then leave bowel in abdomen for 20 minutes surrounded by warm wet packs, then resect ischaemic/non-viable bowel. Do not anastomose bowel at this junction. Leave abdomen open as a laparostomy and bring back to theatre in 24–48 hours when physiologically better with a plan for bowel anastomosis and formal closure.

C Resect bowel where it looks ischaemic. Then if the remaining bowel appears healthy simply re-anastomose it without SMA revascularisation.

D Revascularise the bowel and plan not to resect anything. Leave the abdomen open and aim to bring back in 24–48 hours for formal bowel resection once everything has fully declared itself (*and patient likely in multi-organ failure at this point if the bowel was frankly ischaemic as you opened the patient up*).

E Revascularise the bowel. If the bowel looks ischaemic, then resect it and plan for formal stoma creation and abdominal closure in this sitting.

You open the abdomen. It takes a little longer than usual but you manage to get through the adhesions with no major difficulties. You are confronted with an entirety of small bowel and right colon that looks otherwise well-perfused. It is pink. There is peristalsis visible. There is no free fluid. There is no malodour. The patient has been consented for SMA embolectomy. The root of the mesentery is right in front of you and you are poised to proceed. However, the pH and lactate have improved with some fluid filling (pH 7.31, lactate 1.7, BE −5.5). The anaesthetist remarks that there is some ST depression on the ECG leads which may be exacerbated by mesenteric reperfusion. What are your options here?

✓ A Proceed with SMA embolectomy. This picture may be explained by mucosal small bowel ischaemia that is progressing to trans-mural ischaemia, but you cannot see the external changes. You got the patient transferred to theatre so quickly that you may be falsely reassured at this point by the outer appearance of the bowel.

B Do not proceed with SMA embolectomy. There is the potential to make the bowel considerably worse with embolectomy such as distal propagation into smaller branches with segmental ischaemia +/− SMA dissection. Plan to manage conservatively with further fluid filling, IV heparin, laparostomy, and further re-look in 24 hours (*or sooner if deteriorates*).

C Call interventional radiology to do an on-table angiogram to see what the mesenteric perfusion looks like now with a view to thrombolysis.

D Leave the patient on-table for 3 hours with the vascular registrar scrubbed observing. Go for an extended coffee break. When you come back re-inspect the bowel and decide if you should proceed with an embolectomy or not.

E De-scrub and then run downstairs to the main vascular MDT which is taking place simultaneously. Spend 45 minutes discussing your options (*and likely return still scratching your head*).

CASE REFLECTIONS

Usually, when you go into the abdomen of someone with acute mesenteric ischaemia with raised lactate and acidosis and clot in the SMA you will be met with gut that looks obviously ischaemic. **HOWEVER** – there is a well-known phenomenon that the clinical signs in acute mesenteric ischaemia can be very subtle. Indeed, the classic presentation of acute mesenteric ischaemia is the patient with abdominal pain but very few impressive clinical signs. *Pain out of proportion to the clinical signs* is well known. Indeed, within this clinical context it is only much later on that the patient starts to display signs of peritonism, etc. … but this is when the bowel ischaemia has become trans-mural (*and often if you do a laparotomy at this point the bowel is already dead*).

By way of translating this phenomenon into the operating theatre, there is an argument that if you do a laparotomy on someone with genuine but relatively early acute mesenteric ischaemia, you may visualise the bowel before things have been given the opportunity to fully declare themselves. This is especially the case if you clinch the diagnosis very quickly and get the patient to theatre very quickly. As such, within this context, you may see what looks like "healthy" bowel on the surface, but *the overall picture still suggests something sinister is going on*. In essence, the external appearance of the bowel can be falsely reassuring.

If you do a laparotomy on someone with clot in their SMA and the bowel looks normal, the pH is normal, the lactate is normal, the base excess is normal … I think in this context it is safer to adopt a conservative management approach (*but still remain cautious*). If you do a laparotomy on someone with clot in their SMA and the bowel looks normal, but the pH/lactate/base excess are all abnormal, then the chances are that the inside of the bowel is not healthy. Chances are that you are simply not seeing what is truly going on inside the wall of the gut. If you decide not to revascularise the bowel now (*because it looks completely normal externally*), you may find yourself rushing the patient back to theatre in 12 hours time.

The other thing to mention is that SMA embolectomy/thrombectomy is always going to be a potentially risky and challenging procedure. What you plan to be an SMA embolectomy may actually turn out to be a bit of a nightmare (*such as SMA thromboendarterectomy, patch repair, on-table lysis, patch revision, dissection, need to do an SMA bypass, etc.*). In doing this procedure you definitely can make things worse. Indeed, there are times when there may be genuine equipoise about the pros and cons of mesenteric revascularisation. However, based upon my own experience in this case, I suggest coming back to an appreciation of the overall clinical picture. If the patient has abdominal pain, clot in the main SMA, is showing signs of systemic upset with evidence of malperfusion (*i.e. lactic acidosis*), but the bowel looks externally normal, and I have to get off the fence and make a decision … I would err on the side of mesenteric revascularisation.

Summary Message

- Clot in SMA + abdominal pain + sinister clinical and biochemical signs (*e.g. metabolic acidosis/raised lactate/vomiting/diarrhoea*) + completely normal appearing bowel = SMA embolectomy.

A patient has been assigned to your day-case varicose vein surgery list. This is in a little hospital around 30 minutes away from the main vascular surgery centre. You have not met the patient before, but she has been seen in a one-stop varicose vein clinic by another colleague. You are reading the clinic letter, and determine that:

> This is a 46-year-old female who presents to the outpatient clinic with bilateral symptomatic varicose veins. She is in good general health, is on no regular medications and is allergic to penicillin. There is no history of deep vein thrombosis. On examination there are bilateral, very large varicose veins, extending well up the thigh on both sides. Duplex scanning shows that the varicose veins on the left leg extend to within about 7cm of the saphenofemoral junction where they drain into an incompetent great saphenous vein. There is no short saphenous incompetence and the deep veins look healthy. On the right side the veins drain into an incompetent great saphenous vein.

Based upon the information provided so far, what are your current management considerations for this patient?

  A Conservative management alone.
  B Endovenous laser ablation or radiofrequency ablation with foam sclerotherapy.
  C Endovenous laser ablation or radiofrequency ablation with multiple stab avulsions.
  D Bilateral SFJ ligation, GSV stripping and multiple stab avulsions.
✓ E Potentially all of the above options are possible depending upon subjective opinion.

The clinic letter indicates that the final decision was for open surgical treatment of both legs in the same sitting. On this basis the patient is now sitting in front of you. She is fairly overweight (BMI 42) with very deep groins and a reasonably sized abdominal apron. You first ask the patient what procedure she has come in for today. She informs you that she is expecting only her left leg to be treated. Indeed, the notion of bilateral varicose vein surgery makes her feel nervous. She further explains that her right leg is "not that bad" and it really does not bother her that much. *If* you did agree that varicose vein treatment was justified at this juncture, what would your management plan be now?

  A Politely remind the patient that the clinic letter says she has agreed to both legs being treated, she has been booked for both legs to be treated, and therefore the best approach is to stick to the intended plan.
✓ B Agree to do the left leg alone today and if the right leg needs to be treated in the future we can reassess the situation at a later date.
  C Give the patient the option to have a high tie and strip with avulsions on the left leg, but you can also do avulsions alone on the right leg.
  D Severely reprimand the patient for wasting your time. She has been allocated extra time in theatre to have both legs sorted, and changing the plan now to just one leg will result in wasted theatre time.
  E Change the plan entirely. Inform the patient that you think she is better off with an endovenous approach, and that you think she should be cancelled today, and then brought back to an EVLT list next week.

DOI: 10.1201/9781003497042-10

You and the patient agree to focus on just the left leg today. She is marked and consented for left SFJ ligation, GSV stripping, and multiple stab avulsions. What risks would you include in the consent form?

✓ A Bleeding, infection, wound healing problems, a 1 in 300 risk of provoking a deep vein thrombosis (*with a small risk of progression to a pulmonary embolism*), a 1 in 40 risk of a groin wound infection, a 1 in 20 chance of being left with a patch of numbness, pins and needles, or pain which usually settles but may take several months, and a 10% chance of recurrence of the varicose veins after apparently successful treatment, cosmetic issues, anaesthetic risks, chest infection.

B 1 in 10 risk of a deep vein thrombosis, with the subsequent risk of a fatal pulmonary embolism, recurrence and the need for further procedures, groin complications, infection, bleeding, anaesthetic risks.

C Pain, bleeding, recurrence, further procedures, limb loss, death.

D Recurrence, DVT, PE, chest infection, anaesthetic risks, bleeding, poor cosmetic result.

E Bleeding, infection, neurovascular injury, scarring (*the rest of the risks do not need mentioning as they are already on the clinic letter*).

The patient has arrived in theatre. What would be your standard approach to identifying where to make your groin incision?

A Make your incision in the groin skin crease.

✓ B Use the ultrasound and mark the exact position of the SFJ.

C Vertical groin incision over the femoral artery pulse and then dissect medially to this point.

D Oblique groin incision lateral to the femoral pulse.

E Horizontal 2 cm incision halfway between the anterior superior iliac spine (ASIS) and the pubic tubercle.

Imagine that you have a very proactive and pleasant junior surgical assistant with you today. They turned up at 7.20 am and consented and marked the patient and completed the venous thromboembolism risk assessment. They present the patient to you. They know the relevant anatomy. They explain that they have assisted with this type of procedure before, and have watched some videos and read some book chapters on how the procedure is performed. They ask if they can do the groin dissection.

The patient is positioned supine. You feel obliged to let this trainee do the groin dissection because they are obviously conscientious and pleasant and proactive and keen. You therefore stand on the opposite side of the table while the surgical trainee stands on the ipsilateral groin side. The trainee has the knife in their hand. The dissection continues in a relatively efficient manner down through the layers. Around 20 minutes later the SFJ is fully exposed. You allow the trainee to ligate the SFJ. The stripper is then passed, the GSV is drawn out of the leg, the avulsions proceed, and the groin is closed. The trainee thanks you for being patient with them and then offers to go to the coffee shop downstairs to get you a drink (*which you gratefully accept*). The patient is taken out of theatre into recovery. One minute later the anaesthetist rushes into theatre and asks you to come and see the patient in recovery urgently. Apparently the patient has dropped her blood pressure and there is a very large swelling in the left groin. What do you think the diagnosis is here?

A Iatrogenic common femoral artery injury.

B Small venous tributary is back bleeding.

✓ C Tie has slipped off the SFJ and there is basically major venous bleeding from the common femoral vein.

D Profunda vein must have been avulsed during the original dissection and now it has revealed itself when the patient woke up from general anaesthesia and started moving.

   E The superficial femoral vein must have been accidentally stripped, and the major venous bleeding must be from here.

When you eyeball the patient from the end of the bed she looks pale. There is a very large haematoma in the left groin that is expanding in front of you. The patient's blood pressure is 86/48 mmHg, and the heart rate is 110. The left thigh does not look swollen although it is wrapped up towards the level of the upper thigh. What would be your immediate management plan?

   A Rush the patient back into theatre, do a laparotomy, clamp the infra-renal aorta, resuscitate with IV fluids, then re-open the left groin wound.

✓ B Pressure applied to the left groin. Resuscitate her (*ideally with blood*). Take the patient back to theatre. Re-open the left groin wound but extend your incision medially and laterally. Have some decent suction and retractors available. Plan to compress the CFV above and below the SFJ using your assistants fingers and then properly ***transfix*** the SJF using a heavy vicryl suture.

   C Apply a pressure-dressing to the left groin and tell the anaesthetist and recovery theatre staff to "stop making a mountain out of a molehill". Say you intend to finish your next case, and then after that you will come back to reassess the patient in recovery.

   D Apply a pressure-dressing to the left groin and arrange for immediate transfer to the central vascular surgery unit for a CTA angiogram and venogram +/– covered stenting of the CFV.

   E Open the left groin wound in recovery and prepare to ligate the CFV at the bedside.

The patient is wheeled back into theatre. The anaesthetist has a few units of 0-negative blood available and is putting them up. Someone is pressing over the left groin. You cannot get in contact with your surgical trainee because you do not have their telephone number. Around this same junction, your scrub nurse also faints. What would you do now?

   A Put out a cardiac arrest call for the patient and the scrub nurse.

   B Ask one of the theatre team to look after both the scrub nurse as you go and deal with the patient who is bleeding from the SFJ.

   C Wait until your trainee has returned and then ask them to scrub in and come and assist you.

✓ D Ask one of the theatre team to look after the scrub nurse as you go and deal with the patient who is bleeding from the SFJ. Ask another member of the theatre team to alert the theatre team coordinator as to what is happening, and ask for the coordinator to try and find another surgeon and scrub nurse from an adjacent theatre to come and assist you.

   E Faint yourself.

A surgical registrar from an adjacent theatre comes in to assist you, followed by a urology consultant from another theatre. You all are now scrubbed in together. Another member of your own theatre has already replaced the scrub nurse who fainted. The patient has received 3 units of blood and is much more stable now. The anaesthetist says it is OK for you to proceed as the major transfusion protocol has been activated and all the blood products will be available in around 20 minutes. What would be your management plan now?

✓ A Make a pragmatic decision to proceed ***now***. The notion that the whole "major trauma" blood pack is going to be here in 20 minutes is a fantasy (*you would be pressing on the groin for much longer*). This is not a patient with an aortic injury – it is a tie that has slipped off the SFJ in a groin that has already been dissected. Keep things in perspective therefore. Re-open the groin, get your assistant with a big suction device, and grab the SFJ as quickly as you can with non-toothed forceps to enable it to be transfixed securely.

B Inform the anaesthetist that currently you have control of the bleeding groin simply by compressing it. As soon as you open the groin it is likely going to bleed a lot. It would be better to have the blood products available in theatre and you are ok to wait another 20 minutes.

C Re-open the groin immediately, but have a 1-0 Prolene suture ready. As soon as you can swipe that needle deep into the groin and ligate the entire SFJ/CFV complex (*damage control approach, save life, don't worry about the consequences for the limb*).

D Proceed to a Rutherford Morrison cutdown in the left iliac fossa while someone is pressing in the groin below. Clamp the external iliac vein. Then ask your assistants to apply pressure in the upper thigh to compress the left superficial femoral vein and profunda vein. Once proximal and distal control is achieved you can then re-open the left groin.

E Do a Rutherford Morrison cutdown in the left iliac fossa and flay open the left thigh. This will allow you to fully control the EIV, SFV, and PFV. Then when you have proximal and distal control you can "attack the injury" with a much reduce risk of major bleeding.

You choose option **A**. You open the left groin and there is profuse/torrential haemorrhage pouring straight up at you. You ask the surgical registrar to suck the blood away whilst the urology consultant presses the upper thigh using his hand (*to compress the deep veins distal to your wound*) whilst he uses his fingers to compress the CFV above the bleeding point. You can see the SFJ and quickly grab it with some non-toothed forceps. You quickly transfix it using 2-0 vicryl, washout the groin, and then close the groin. You ask the anaesthetist to give some appropriate IV antibiotics to reduce the risk of surgical site infection. You thank your assistants who then go back to what they were doing.

Around 3 minutes after completing this operation, your surgical trainee walks back into theatre with a very pale look on their face. They have your coffee in their hand. They apologise profusely for being absent but they had just finished their lunch and had no idea what was happening in theatre.

CASE REFLECTIONS

This is ***not*** a real case and it does not reflect routine practice, however there are elements of truth interspersed throughout the case. The case is designed to highlight pitfalls and red flags and worst-case scenarios. It also highlights some of the practicalities related to day-case varicose vein surgery in remote hospitals. The few areas I wish to focus on are:

1) Pushing surgical boundaries.
2) Classic pitfalls in open varicose vein surgery.
3) Recognising where you are and what surgical assistance you have available.
4) Dealing with bleeding in a pragmatic and realistic manner.
5) Having a really bad day summary.

Pushing Surgical Boundaries

A slim fit patient with a "virgin" groin is a great open varicose vein surgery case. The exposure and dissection are relatively easy, and it is also the ideal training case for a junior surgeon. However, if this is the ideal open varicose vein surgery case, there are patients on the other end of the spectrum. These are the comorbid obese patients with bilateral massive varicose veins and re-do groins. Notice in this case that I deliberately ascribed our patient a BMI of 42 to make such a point about pushing boundaries.

In regard to pushing boundaries, I would simply recommend maintaining overall insight. Vascular surgery as a whole can be as easy and as difficult *as you decide*. I do not mind a challenge, but there is a difference between a challenge and making your life unnecessarily difficult (*and arguably more dangerous for the patient*). Varicose vein surgery will always carry risks, but prolonged complex re-do surgery in an obese comorbid patient will naturally increase the risks of bleeding, surgical site infection, venous thromboembolism and likely varicose vein recurrence. Something for you (*and me*) to reflect upon.

Classic Pitfalls in Open Varicose Vein Surgery

I do not know all of them but these are the main ones I am aware of (*folklore probably*):

- Tie slipping off the SJF (*I always transfix it*).
- Stripping the superficial femoral vein instead of the GSV (*I always make sure I can see the CFV above and below the SFJ to be absolutely certain*).
- Injuring the deep external pudendal artery at the SFJ/CFV junction.
- Losing the stripper in the leg (*I always tie it to a heavy vicryl reel*).
- Injuring the CFV during re-do varicose vein surgery. I always remember that a re-do groin dissection is important to do properly, but not at the expense of causing major deep venous bleeding. I guess my advice would be to maintain insight and exercise discretion with how aggressive you think you should be in skeletonising the CFV.
- Being so carefree about your avulsions that you do not realise that you have already lost 4 units of blood. Press on the avulsions sites afterwards do not just let them bleed and bleed and bleed!

Recognising Where You Are and What Surgical Assistance You Have Available

In my practice most open varicose vein surgery is performed in a little hospital a few miles away from the main vascular centre. Other day-case surgery like hernia repairs, lump and bump excisions, and minor urology procedures are often taking place in adjacent theatres. As such, there is often a little mixture of vascular surgeons, plastic surgeons, general surgeons, and urologists around in daylight hours. There might be another vascular surgeon downstairs doing an outpatient clinic. However, this centre does not do major arterial surgery and the set-up is not geared for this. There is not a massive blood bank. There is not an ICU. There is no interventional radiology on-site.

I mention this because if you were to encounter a vascular complication in this sort of setting you will likely not get the equipment and assistance/support you would normally expect if you were back in the main vascular centre. Also, having loads of blood products (*i.e. the classic 1:1:1 trauma mix of blood, fresh frozen plasma and platelets*) may be a luxury you simply do not have (*or will not have in a timely fashion*). It may also be that if you are in a hospital that is really quite far away from the main vascular centre calling for help may not be of much use in the moment (*because it would take too long for someone to arrive*). This theatre set-up is not "wrong," it just means that you have to risk assess which patients and operations you are going to perform in such a setting.

Dealing with Bleeding in a Pragmatic and Realistic Manner

If a patient has a hosing groin because of a major arterial injury, then I would manage this with a standard "proximal and distal control" approach, i.e. probably Rutherford Morrison incision and then a fairly extensive upper thigh incision to expose the SFA/PFA, etc. However, the case described above simply has slipped SFJ tie written all over it. The groin dissection has already been done. All you really need to do is open the groin very quickly, suck the blood out of the way, and get your assistant to press below on the thigh to slow down the bleeding own enough to allow you to grab the SFJ with some non-toothed forceps. This likely will be a bit juicy for around 30 seconds, but it should not be too laborious and the blood loss should not be too significant. As such, in my opinion, I think the option **A** approach seems fairly reasonable within this specific context. Doing a full Rutherford Morrison incision, flaying open the thigh and waiting around for 30–45 minutes for the whole trauma blood transfusion package to be delivered just feels like overkill to me. Furthering this theme, I also question how much benefit there is in calling for senior vascular surgery assistance. If I know there is a vascular consultant in the outpatient department downstairs then this is definitely what I would do, but if I knew I was on my own I would just be realistic and see if there was another helpful colleague next door. General surgeons and plastic surgeons and urologists are perfectly capable of providing suitable assistance in such a setting, and they would be more helpful to me than a vascular surgery consultant who is going to take an hour to get here.

Having a Really Bad Day Summary

The notion of the trainee being unintentionally absent and the scrub nurse fainting was included mainly to morph this case further into being a worst-case scenario. This is a very uncommon occurrence. However, this possibility is worth considering because Sod's law would dictate that if this sort of thing were to happen, it would likely happen at the worst possible time! Also, continuing this theme of life not being fair – if you are truly in **big trouble** (*i.e. bad bleeding that demands you do something about it fairly quickly*) but there is no CT or interventional radiology available, there are no other vascular surgeons around, your assistant has disappeared, and there is very limited blood available … you may find this simplistic bleeding algorithm below helpful (*Figure 10.1*). The most important thing in a scenario like this is to try and stay calm and stay cool – if you start panicking and losing your cool everybody else in theatre is likely to start panicking and losing their cool (*and this is probably what majorly contributes to scrub nurses fainting, which is clearly not what you need*).

KEEP A COOL HEAD

STAY CALM

ONE

Apply pressure and try to achieve at least proximal control

Consider using a tourniquet if you suspect an arterial bleed and you can get above the bleeding point

Consider compressing common femoral artery in groin

FOUR

Return to theate ASAP

Try to keep things simple, and stick to core vascular surgery principles

SIGNIFICANT POST-OPERATIVE LOWER LIMB BLEEDING

Expanding haematoma
Visual profuse bleeding
Surgical drain filled up rapidly
Haemodynamic instability
Patient looks white etc...

TWO

Call for help

When time is short remember that a non-vascular surgeon who is closeby and willing and able is better than a vascular surgeon who is an hour away!

THREE

Resuscitation

If someone is bleeding and unstable they ideally should get blood (old fashioned 0-ve probably)
If the systolic BP is >70mmHg, the conscious level is intact, it is difficult to compress the bleeding point, and there is limited blood available, you may have to initially pursue a permissive hypotension approach and use blood sparingly (but obviously try and get blood and blood products to you ASAP)

Figure 10.1 Really bad day post-op lower limb bleeding algorithm.

CASE 11: CHRONIC LIMB-THREATENING ISCHAEMIA

A 65-year-old male presents to your vascular surgery outpatient clinic with dry gangrene to his left third toe, along with severe rest pain and night pain and some ischaemic ulceration to his adjacent toes. He has an extensive vascular surgery history (*that spans many many years and includes procedures performed in another vascular department … frankly I am struggling to recount everything he has had done because it is very complicated and extensive, and much more than what I include below*):

- Bilateral iliac angioplasties/stents.
- Subsequent aorto-bifemoral bypass when the iliacs re-occluded.
- This aorto-bifemoral bypass became infected and required explantation.
- Following this he required a right axillo-popliteal bypass, but this occluded resulting in a right above-knee amputation.
- Subsequent left iliac endovascular recannalisation.
- Subsequent left SFA occlusion recannalisation (*which then occluded*).
- Now chronic left SFA occlusion that has been managed conservatively for the past few years.

The patient says that his left foot pain is so severe that he can barely sleep, and he has to hang his left leg out of bed at night. He has not had a myocardial infarction or a stroke before. He is known to have chronic obstructive pulmonary disease (COPD), but according to him, it is not that bad. He is no longer smoking. He is already on the best medical therapy (clopidogrel 75 mg 0D & atorvastatin 80 mg 0D). On examination he is very thin with very little body fat. He has no pulses in the left leg. He has a right radial pulse. He has a left radial pulse.

See the image of the patient's previous MRA (*from 12 months ago – Figure 11.1*). What do you make of it?

A Patent infra-renal aorta. Patent left iliac system. Long SFA occlusion. Satisfactory popliteal reforms. High PT take-off otherwise good 3-vessel run-off.

B Patent infra-renal aorta. Patent left iliac system but some proximal common iliac disease. Long SFA occlusion. Satisfactory popliteal reforms with normal 3-vessel run-off.

✓ C Patent infra-renal aorta. Patent left iliac system but some proximal common iliac disease. Long SFA occlusion. Satisfactory popliteal reforms. High PT take-off otherwise good 3-vessel run-off.

D Patent infra-renal aorta. Patent iliac system but severely diseased left external iliac. Short SFA occlusion. Diseased popliteal reforms. High PT take-off otherwise good 3-vessel run-off.

E Patent infra-renal aorta. Occluded left iliac system. Long SFA occlusion. Satisfactory popliteal reforms. High PT take-off otherwise good 3-vessel run-off.

What is your initial management plan for this patient?

A Lower limb arterial duplex.

✓ B CT angiogram or MR angiogram lower limbs.

C Palliative care referral.

D List for left high above-knee amputation.

E List for left iliac recannalisation (again).

DOI: 10.1201/9781003497042-11

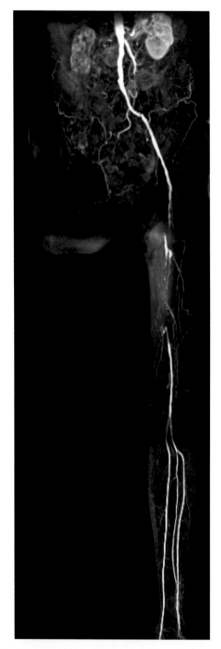

Figure 11.1   Previous MR angiogram lower limbs.

What do you make of the CT angiogram images (see Figures 11.2 and 11.3)?

 A Occluded infra-renal aorta. Occluded left iliac system and left superficial femoral artery. Patent distal left profunda femoris artery. Recannalisation of the popliteal artery at the adductor hiatus with 3-vessel run-off.

✓ B Occluded infra-renal aorta. Occluded left iliac system and left superficial femoral artery. Patent but small distal left profunda femoris artery. Recannalisation of the popliteal artery at the adductor hiatus but diseased behind the knee. Three-vessel run-off.

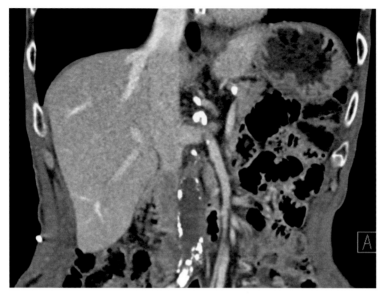

Figure 11.2   CT angiogram image of infra-renal aorta.

C Patent infra-renal aorta. Occluded left iliac system and left superficial femoral artery. Patent but small distal left profunda femoris artery. Recannalisation of the popliteal artery at the adductor hiatus but diseased behind the knee. Three-vessel run-off.

D Patent infra-renal aorta. Occluded left iliac system and left superficial femoral artery. Occluded left profunda artery. Recannalisation of the popliteal artery at the adductor hiatus but diseased behind the knee. Three-vessel run-off.

E Occluded infra-renal aorta. Occluded left iliac system, diseased but patent superficial femoral artery. Patent but small distal left profunda femoris artery. Recannalisation of the popliteal artery at the adductor hiatus. Three-vessel run-off.

What are some potentially viable left leg revascularisation options?

A Right to left femoral-femoral crossover.

B Right to left femoral-femoral crossover and then femoral-AK popliteal bypass.

C Infra-renal aortic thromboendarterectomy, re-do aorto-femoral bypass, then fem-AK popliteal bypass.

✓ D Left axillo-profunda-popliteal bypass.

E Left aortoiliac stenting followed by left fem-BK popliteal artery bypass.

What do you make of the vein mapping result (Figure 11.4)?

A Could do a left axillo-profunda-popliteal bypass using spliced basilic vein and left GSV.

B Could do a left axillo-profunda bypass using spliced basilic vein and above-knee amputation.

C Could do a left axillo-profunda prosthetic bypass and then a profunda-popliteal bypass using spliced basilic vein.

✓ D Could do a left axillo-profunda-popliteal bypass using two prosthetic bypasses with left calf GSV vein cuff/s.

E Could do a left axillo-profunda-popliteal bypass using spliced cephalic and basilic vein.

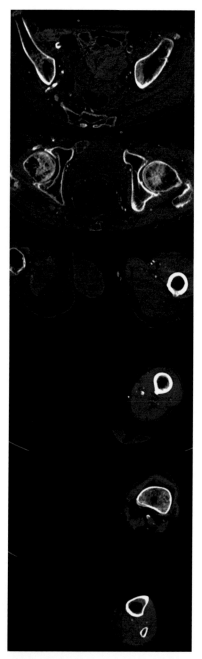

Figure 11.3   CT angiogram lower limbs.

The position of the vascular MDT after reviewing the CTA is that the only options available are:

- Left axillo-profunda-popliteal bypass.
- Left axillo-profunda bypass and above-knee amputation.
- Palliation.

Clinical indication - all studies

ortic occlusion + SFA disease of remaining LLL. ?revascularisation options

Lower limb vein map - Left

No true SFJ, ? Previous surgery. There is a small calibre vein at the groin ? Source, this vein can be traced caudally with an appearance of an LSV within the thigh, in the distal thigh the vein branches and communicates with a vein within the calf. The ? LSV can be followed throughout the calf branching in the mid calf.

? LSV proximal thigh - 2.5mm
? LSV mid thigh - 3.3mm
? LSV distal thigh -1.8mm
LSV proximal calf - 5mm
LSV mid calf - 4.6mm
LSV distal calf - 4.5mm

Upper limb vein map - Right

The cephalic vein is a good calibre in the forearm, draining directly into the large basilic vein at the ACF. Small calibre cephalic vein cranial to the elbow. The confluence of the basilic vein is high in the proximal humerus, good length.

Cephalic vein (mid humerus) - 1.3mm

Cephalic vein (distal humerus) - 1.1mm
Cephalic vein (proximal forearm) - 3.1mm
Cephalic vein (mid forearm) - 3.3mm
Cephalic vein (distal forearm) - 2.1mm
Basilic Vein - (distal humerus) 6.5 mm
Basilic Vein - (mid humerus) 6.2 mm
Basilic Vein -(proximal humerus) 6.1 mm

Upper limb vein map - Left

The cephalic vein is smaller in the forearm compared to the right. The Cephalic vein throughout the humerus is small in calibre. The cephalic vein communicates with the basilic vein at the ACF via a branch vessel. Good calibre basilic vein with its confluence in the proximal humerus.

Cephalic vein (mid humerus) - 1.1mm
Cephalic vein (distal humerus) - 1.7mm
Cephalic vein (proximal forearm) - .3mm
Cephalic vein (mid forearm) - 2.1mm
Cephalic vein (distal forearm) - 2.1mm
Basilic Vein - (distal humerus) 4.6 mm
Basilic Vein - (mid humerus) 6.1 mm
Basilic Vein -(proximal humerus) 4.5 mm

Figure 11.4   Vein mapping result.

The patient is adamant that he does not want to lose his left leg, nor does he want to be palliated. He wishes to proceed with an attempt at limb salvage, i.e. left axillo-profunda-popliteal bypass. What are some things you would want to confirm before proceeding with such a case?

A Patient has up-to-date echocardiogram and pulmonary function tests, anaesthetic review, and left axillary artery duplex to confirm there is a decent inflow source.

B Patient has up-to-date echocardiogram and pulmonary function tests, anaesthetic review, left axillary artery duplex to confirm there is a decent inflow source, patient has been thoroughly counselled on the risks and benefits of the proposed procedure, and his family is on board with the plan.

C Patient has up-to-date echocardiogram and pulmonary function tests, anaesthetic review, left axillary artery duplex to confirm there is a decent inflow source, patient has been thoroughly counselled on the risks and benefits of the proposed procedure, his family is on board with the plan, that you have suitable grafts available for this case, that you have scrutinised the run-off vessels as per his previous imaging, and that you will have a suitable (*i.e. senior*) surgical assistance for the case.

D Patient has up-to-date echocardiogram and pulmonary function tests, anaesthetic review, left axillary artery duplex to confirm there is a decent inflow source, patient has been thoroughly counselled on the risks and benefits of the proposed procedure, his family is on board with the plan, that you have suitable grafts available for this case, that you have scrutinised the run-off vessels as per his previous imaging, and that you will have a suitable (*i.e. senior*) surgical assistance for the case, and that you have the support of the intensive care team.

✓ E Patient has up-to-date echocardiogram and pulmonary function tests, anaesthetic review, left axillary artery duplex to confirm there is a decent inflow source, patient has been thoroughly counselled on the risks and benefits of the proposed procedure, his family is on board with the plan, that you have suitable infection-resistant grafts available for this case, that you have scrutinised the run-off vessels as per his previous imaging, and that you will have a suitable (*i.e. senior*) surgical assistance for the case, and that you have the support of the intensive care team.

Please review the following fitness test results (Figure 11.5). Do you think this patient sounds like a viable open surgical candidate?

A Heart is OK. Lungs are as expected. Kidneys are OK. This patient has survived every other vascular operation. He doesn't want to lose his leg, and he doesn't want to die. Why not?

B These tests are reassuring, but this surgery seems very unlikely to be successful, and therefore I just don't think it is viable.

C These tests are reassuring, but the risk of infection is just too high; therefore, I just don't think it is viable.

D These tests are reassuring, but the patient is so thin and his albumin is a bit low; therefore, I think that his wounds will all break down, and I just don't think it is viable.

✓ E Heart is OK. Lungs are as expected. Kidneys are OK. This patient has survived every other vascular operation. He doesn't want to lose his leg, and he doesn't want to die. He appears to have decent run-off. If he has a decent left axillary artery on duplex I think this case is fair game … but I am going to try and get some infection-resistant grafts and make sure I cover the groin anastomoses with a muscle flap.

Transthoracic Echocardiogram

Conclusion:
Normal bi-ventricular function. Estimated LVEF 55-60%.
Mild to moderate TR.

Reported by:	**Angus Meikle**
Signed by:	**Angus Meikle**
Date Signed:	**01/02/2024 10:34AM**

Spirometry

Substance		Pred LL	Pred	Meas	% Pred	Z-Score
Dose						
FEV 1	L	2.50	3.48	1.80	51.9	-2.74
FVC	L	3.44	4.64	3.28	70.7	-1.86
FEV 1 % FVC	%	61.96	75.38	54.94	72.9	-2.41
PEF	L/min	391	510	421	82.6	-1.22
MFEF 75/25	L/s	1.11	2.57	0.61	23.8	-2.45
FEF 50 % MIF 50	%			70.95		
VC MAX	L	3.97	4.99	3.28	65.8	-2.78

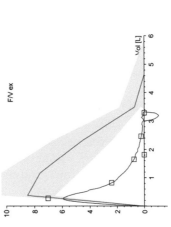

Full blood Count FBC

Result	Value	Units	Ref. Range
Haemoglobin	166	g/L	135-180
White cell count	6.02	10^9/L	4.00-11.00
Platelets	203	10^9/L	150-400

Clotting Screen

Result	Value	Units	Ref. Range
Prothrombin time	12	s	9-14
INR (p=poc)	1.0		
Derived Fibrinogen	>4.5	g/L	1.6-5.9
APTT (a=anticoag therapy)	34.5	s	23.5-37.5
APTT Ratio (a=anticoag therapy)	1.1		0.8-1.2
Set Comment:	High Fibrinogen results may indicate		

Urea & Electrolytes

Result	Value	Units	Ref. Range
Sodium	138	mmol/L	133-146
Potassium	3.8	mmol/L	3.5-5.3
Urea	7.8	mmol/L	2.5-7.8
Creatinine	65	umol/L	64-104
eGFR	>90	mL/min/1.73m2	
Set Comment:	Interpret eGFR with caution in adults suspected, please REPEAT serum cr		

CRP

Result	Value	Units	Ref. Range
CRP	8.6	mg/L	<10.0

Liver Function Test

Result	Value	Units	Ref. Range
Bilirubin	7	umol/L	2-21
ALT	16	iu/L	<40
Albumin	33	g/L	35-50
Alk Phos	83	iu/L	30-130

Figure 11.5 Fitness test results.

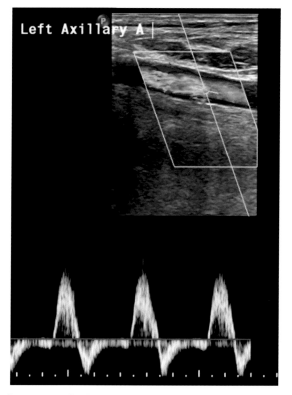

Figure 11.6 Left axillary artery duplex.

What do you make of this left axillary artery duplex (Figure 11.6)?

    A Triphasic flow and disease-free axillary artery – game on.

✓ B Biphasic flow in a slightly calcified axillary artery – game on.

    C Monophasic flow – game over.

    D Biphasic flow just ain't good enough for me to take on a case like this. I need perfection (i.e. triphasic flow).

    E Monophasic flow – game on.

You seemingly have a reasonable left axillary artery to use as an inflow source. Based upon the imaging of the run-off vessels, what do you think is the best target vessel for your distal anastomosis at the knee?

✓ A Posterior tibial artery in the below-knee segment (*accepting this is a high posterior tibial artery take-off as per the MRA*).

    B Above-knee popliteal artery.

    C Anterior tibial artery.

    D Peroneal artery.

    E Below-knee popliteal artery just above the origin of the anterior tibial artery.

The patient ultimately went on to have a left axillary-upper thigh profunda artery bypass with a silver-coated antibiotic-impregnated ring-enforced 8 mm graft and ipsilateral GSV Miller cuff, and a jump graft to the posterior tibial artery with a silver-coated antibiotic-impregnated ring-enforced 6 mm graft and ipsilateral GSV miller cuff, with sartorius flap coverage.

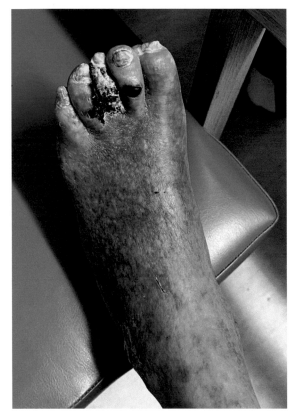

Figure 11.7 Left foot pre-operatively.

How would you have exposed the left profunda artery?

A Re-do vertical groin cutdown (through old scar), fully expose CFA, then chase downwards to expose the origin of the PFA and go distally.

✓ B Incision from the anterior superior iliac spine (ASIS) swung obliquely across the left groin and down the thigh. Expose the medial border of sartorius and lift it laterally. Expose virgin SFA underneath the sartorius muscle distal to the scarred groin, sloop it, lift it medially, and then find virgin PFA directly underneath the SFA. At the end of the operation the sartorius can be disconnected from the ASIS and used as a flap to cover your anastomoses and grafts.

C Mark out the profunda artery in the upper thigh using ultrasound and try and find it that way.

D Mark out the SFA in the upper thigh using ultrasound, then find the profunda artery underneath the SFA in virgin territory.

E Just make a big cut in the groin and dissect in multiple different planes until you find something vaguely resembling the profunda artery (*but preferably don't anastomose onto the femoral nerve*).

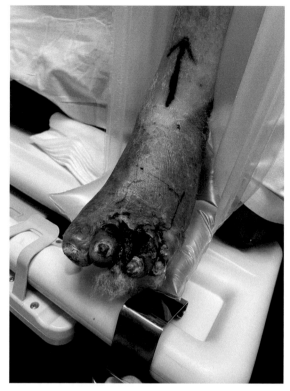

Figure 11.8   Left foot post-operatively.

If this was what the foot looked like pre-op (Figure 11.7), what should you be specifically wary of post-operatively (*if you bypass was successful*)?

   A Compartment syndrome.

   B Reperfusion oedema.

✓ C Reperfusion foot sepsis.

   D Graft infection.

   E Cardiac arrhythmias.

Post-operatively the patient has a strong biphasic PT signal using the handheld Doppler and the patient develops obvious reperfusion oedema to the foot. The left forefoot also deteriorates and becomes wet with minor forefoot cellulitis. What would be your management plan in this context (see Figure 11.8)?

   A Oral antibiotics.

   B Intravenous antibiotics.

   C Intravenous antibiotics and left forefoot amputation (*with above-knee tourniquet used to minimise blood loss*).

   D Left below-knee amputation.

✓ E Intravenous antibiotics and left forefoot amputation.

See some relevant operative images in Figures 11.9, 11.10, 11.11, and 11.12.

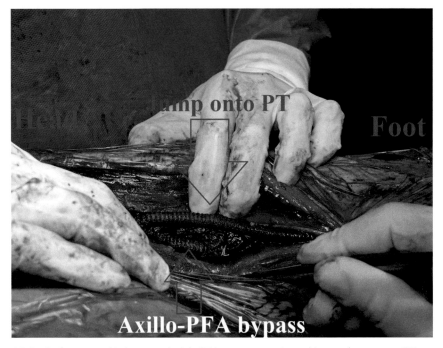

Figure 11.9 Left upper thigh wound with PFA anastomosis and jump down onto PT.

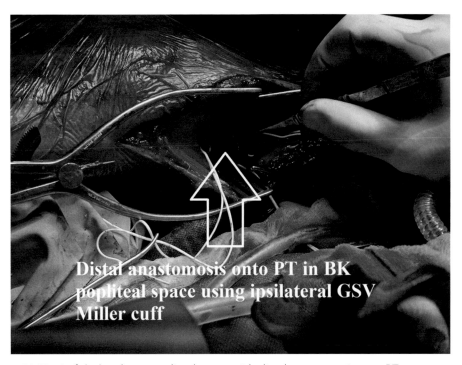

Figure 11.10 Left below-knee popliteal space with distal anastomosis onto PT.

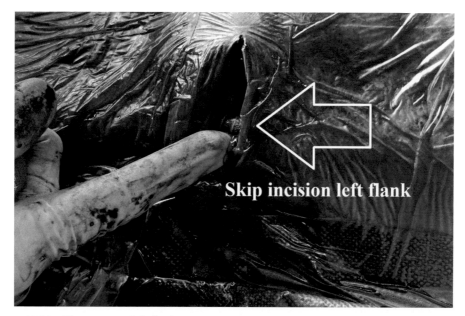

Figure 11.11   Skip incision left flank.

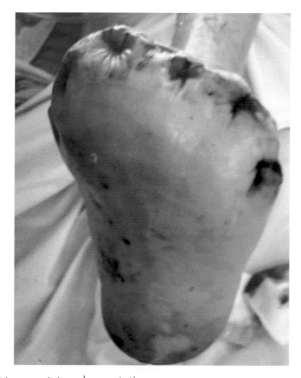

Figure 11.12   Left transmetatarsal amputation.

CASE REFLECTIONS

I vividly recall this patient being discussed in a vascular MDT around one week before I was invited to do his operation. At the time of the MDT discussion, it seemed that such a revascularisation proposal was unusual and challenging and possibly pessimistic, to say the least. Indeed, of all the patients I have ever seen who have had an axillary-PFA-popliteal bypass, I had seen them *years after* it had already occluded. The other options on the table were not better however i.e. a palliative approach or a high above-knee amputation without inflow correction or an above-knee amputation with an axillary-profunda bypass. As is predictable in vascular surgery, the patient did not want to lose his leg, and he did not want to die either.

I did not like the look of his vein map result and the notion of using spliced basilic vein of probably insufficient length just seemed to be making a difficult and long operation even more difficult and long. Some surgeons may have used spliced vein or taken the ipsilateral distal calf GSV for the profunda-PT bypass, and this is theoretically an acceptable alternative. However, having seen this patient from the end of the bed, I did not think he was the sort of patient who I wanted on-table for very long. Frankly, using vein for him would have resulted in more upper limb wounds or a much longer ipsilateral distal calf wound, more bleeding, more time in theatre, more risk of wound infection and wound breakdown- my instinct simply deterred me from using vein and shunted me instead into being a pragmatist and using prosthetic for everything. Indeed, sometimes surgical decisions are based upon pragmatism and instinct. I was also not too happy with the popliteal artery behind the knee either, and thought it was the PT that was the better vessel below the knee. Although he had a decent left radial pulse, I wanted to further "tick the box" and have a formal arterial duplex that demonstrated that his left axillary artery was of acceptable quality. Finally, I wanted to make sure that the general approach here was one of exhaustively trying to minimise the infection risk, so we pulled out all the stops i.e. everybody washed their hands, used the scrubber on their fingernails, double surgical prep, Ioban, infection-resistant grafts, and muscle flap coverage. The inclusion of two GSV Miller cuffs was as advised from another vascular surgery consultant colleague i.e. this patient had one shot at a successful outcome, so you might as well do everything to maximise the chances of the bypass outflow being decent.

I had also seen the patient in CLTI clinic and counselled him extensively, reinforcing that this was fairly unusual surgery and it had no guarantee of success. I did highlight, however, that his other options were not great either: a left high above-knee amputation (*which may not heal as he had no inflow*), a left axillary-PFA bypass and above-knee amputation (*which would likely result in his axillary-PFA bypass occluding early and his AKA subsequently not healing*), or palliation. The patient had already decided before seeing me that he did not want to die nor lose his leg. He understood the complication profile (*having experienced such complications many times before*), he was of the attitude that he had got through all the other numerous major vascular surgery operations and had survived, and he thought that he was stuck between a rock and a hard place anyways … he was therefore completely in support of the proposed revascularisation plan. His family also supported his decision. I made sure that the rationale for the decision-making (i.e. the risks/benefits/alternatives) and the patient counselling process was documented thoroughly in the medical notes.

The surgery proceeded as expected and it was actually quite easy as the patient was so slim. We stayed away from his re-do groin and simply exposed the PFA is virgin territory lower down the thigh (*underneath the sartorius and SFA*). We used ipsilateral calf GSV to create two Miller cuffs for use on the PFA and PT. Post-operatively the patient had a fantastic biphasic PT signal at the ankle. He developed significant reperfusion oedema. He also developed reperfusion sepsis in the forefoot and ended up needed a left transmetatarsal amputation. This transmetatarsal amputation bled very well (*which is good*). The forefoot amputation wound healed and the patient went home to make a good recovery (*with his leg intact*).

Subjectively from the outset, it seemed like a case that was more likely to be unsuccessful than successful. However, at the same time, why wouldn't it be successful? He had a decent inflow source, we used some infection-resistant grafts that bypassed onto decent outflow vessels with the help of some vein cuffs, the groin plumbing was covered with a viable sartorius muscle flap, and he was actually objectively fit (*i.e. decent echo, reasonable lungs, decent kidneys*).

Main Learning Points

- Successful bypass surgery (*on the whole*) = acceptably and pragmatically fit patient (*mainly heart, lungs and kidneys, if you are expecting an Olympic athlete you need to start living in the real world*) + acceptable inflow + acceptable conduit + acceptable outflow + acceptable resistance to infection.
- If you can somehow tick all of the above boxes, I say **GAME ON** (*i.e. perfection is the enemy of good*).
- If you are going to perform complex and unusual surgery where the stakes are high, make sure that the "risk/benefit/alternative profile" naturally directs itself to your chosen surgical procedure, the patient and family are on board, the vascular MDT and your colleagues are on board, your documentation is excellent, and you have maximised your chances of surgical success.
- Autologous vein is the ideal conduit for distal bypass surgery especially when there is tissue loss in the foot. However, in some cases for pragmatic purposes you may decide to use prosthetic instead, and using prosthetic is not necessarily the wrong decision within certain contexts. You simply have to be able to justify your decision-making and probably anticipate another surgeon saying that they would have used vein. When it comes to the crunch what you are really looking for is a 1) live patient 2) with a bypass that is working and 3) infection-free and 4) wounds that have not broken down and 5) a leg that will remain attached. *How you achieve this arguably sits within the realm of the phrase "horses for courses."*

CASE 12: CAROTID

The wife of a 74-year-old male dials for an ambulance because her husband is struggling to speak and has new right arm weakness whilst he is sitting on the sofa at home. This is on a background of right arm numbness "on and off" lasting only seconds on a few occasions over the last week. By the time the ambulance arrives the symptoms have almost fully resolved. What is your first impression?

   A Stroke.

✓ B Transient ischaemic attack(s).

   C Seizure activity.

   D Migraine.

   E Functional symptoms.

The patient's past medical history includes angina and hypertension. He is on aspirin and low-dose statin therapy. He is an ex-smoker. He is otherwise independent. When the patient is first assessed by a member of the stroke team in A&E he has minimal expressive dysphasia for occasional words, but he can name a lot of common objects. There is now no right arm weakness (power is 5/5) with normal sensation. What do you think would be an appropriate management strategy at this junction?

   A Immediate thrombolysis.

✓ B CT head.

   C Commence on dual antiplatelet therapy and high-dose statin therapy, then discharge home.

   D MRI head.

   E Carotid duplex.

The patient has a CT head. The initial report states no acute intra-cranial abnormality. An amended report 2 hours later says: "*Left MCA appears mildly denser than the right side which suggests potential thrombus.*" The stroke team had initially decided against thrombolysis as the patient's symptoms were deemed too mild. What do you think is the next appropriate step for this patient?

✓ A Routine bloods including HBA1c and lipid screen. ECG. Commence on dual antiplatelet therapy and high-dose statin therapy. Carotid duplex.

   B Thrombolysis.

   C Routine bloods including HBA1c and lipid screen. Commence on oral anticoagulation if ECG normal, along with high-dose statin therapy.

   D Routine bloods including HBA1c and lipid screen. ECG. Commence on dual antiplatelet therapy and high-dose statin therapy. MRA carotids.

   E Routine bloods including HBA1c and lipid screen. ECG. Commence on dual antiplatelet therapy and high-dose statin therapy. Diagnostic angiogram of carotids and circle of Willis.

DOI: 10.1201/9781003497042-12

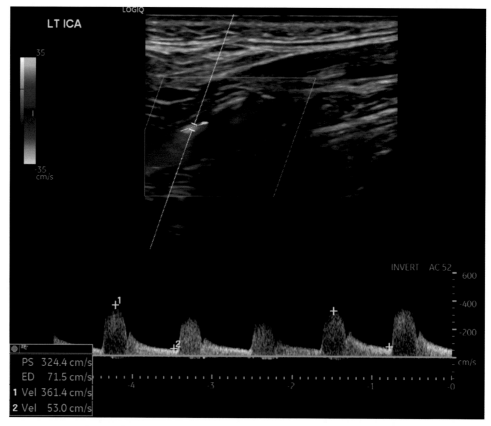

Figure 12.1 Left ICA duplex.

The patient is commenced upon clopidogrel in addition to his usual aspirin, along with high-dose statin therapy. His ECG is normal (*i.e. sinus rhythm*). What is your interpretation of the carotid duplex image (Figure 12.1)?

   A Significant left ICA stenosis.
   B Moderate left ICA stenosis.
   C 50% left ICA stenosis.
   D Insignificant left ICA stenosis.
✓ E 70–89% left ICA stenosis (*somewhere in this ballpark, anyways*).

If this was deemed to be a significant left ICA stenosis, what would be your provisional management plan for this patient?

   A Best medical therapy.
   B Best medical therapy and for primary consideration of carotid stenting.
   C Best medical therapy and for primary consideration of carotid endarterectomy.
✓ D Best medical therapy, for primary consideration of carotid endarterectomy, and if so for dual imaging.
   E Best medical therapy, for primary consideration of carotid stenting, and if so for dual imaging.

What factors would influence your decision-making in regard to suitability for carotid endarterectomy or carotid stenting?

A Patient factors (*femoral pulse status, scars in neck, range of movement of neck, previous radiotherapy to neck, thickness and length of neck*), evidence, guidelines, accessibility of the lesion on imaging, MDT consensus, patient preference.

B MDT consensus.

C Stroke team opinion.

D Patient factors (*femoral pulse status, scars in neck, range of movement of neck, previous radiotherapy to neck, thickness and length of neck*), evidence, guidelines, accessibility of the lesion on imaging, MDT consensus.

✓ E Patient factors (*femoral pulse status, scars in neck, range of movement of neck, previous radiotherapy to neck, thickness and length of neck*), evidence, guidelines, accessibility of the lesion on imaging, vascular MDT consensus, stroke team opinion, patient preference.

The patient has easily palpable femoral pulses. He has a long thin neck with an excellent range of movement. He has no scars in his neck, and no reports of previous radiotherapy to the neck. He also has now had some further imaging of his carotids (Figure 12.2). What is your opinion on this additional information?

A Seems like an excellent candidate for carotid stenting.

B Seems like an appropriate candidate for right carotid endarterectomy.

✓ C Seems like an appropriate candidate for left carotid endarterectomy.

D Seems like an excellent candidate for left carotid endarterectomy, but will definitely require a shunt and therefore must be performed under general anaesthetic.

E The carotid is occluded; therefore, carotid endarterectomy is not appropriate.

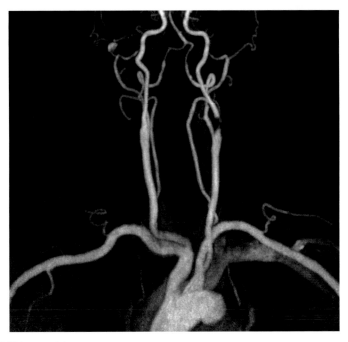

Figure 12.2 MRA carotids.

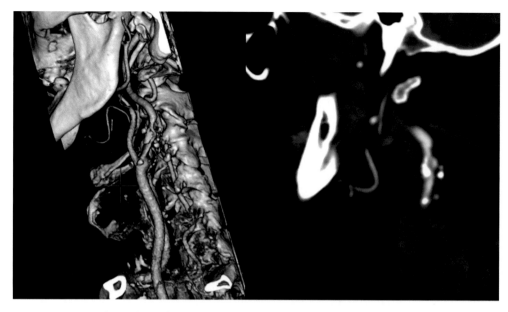

L ICA stenosis, recent R hemispheric event   Looks to be possible high
bifurcation on MR. CTA please ?high bifurcation (above C3 endplate) for risk stratiofication

Report Body - CT Angio aortic arch & carotid Both

Comparison made to previous MRA

Patent left common carotid artery with the bifurcation demonstrated at the superior end plate of C4, below the level of the mandible. Severe stenosis of the left ICA from its origin up to the formation of the horizontal segment, approximately 60-70% on CT. The remainder of the ICA is patent, no tandem lesion. Patent left ECA.

Patent right innominate artery. Patent right common carotid artery. No significant right ICA stenosis. The remainder of the ICA is patent. Patent right ECA.

Comments: 60-70% left ICA stenosis.

Figure 12.3   Further CTA carotids to confirm it was a high lesion.

The MRA report states that this is a severe left ICA stenosis of (>90%). Just because you are having a lucky day (*this isn't normal practice but there were some concerns about the quality of the MRA and how high the ICA lesion was*), the patient also had another form of vascular imaging of his carotid vessels (Figure 12.3).

The patient is appropriately counselled and would like to proceed with carotid endarterectomy. *If, however,* the patient had previously had an operation in the anterior triangle of his right neck, what would your management plan be in this specific context?

  A Carotid endarterectomy is contraindicated. Proceed with carotid stenting.
✓ B Carotid endarterectomy is not absolutely contraindicated, but the patient requires an indirect laryngoscopy to ensure there are no vocal cord issues. If there is a contralateral vocal cord palsy, the indication for carotid endarterectomy should be seriously reconsidered.
  C There are no issues because the previous operation was on the contralateral side. Proceed with left carotid endarterectomy.
  D Do not proceed with any surgical or endovascular carotid intervention. Manage the patient by way of best medical therapy alone.
  E Wait for 3 months and then proceed with carotid stenting.

Imagine that you have never seen this patient before, and he has been listed for a carotid end-arterectomy by another surgeon. The patient is assigned to your operation list however. When the patient arrives on the day of surgery you go to see him. You discover that what is documented in the medical notes is not actually what you now find in the "real world." For example, the patient is not on the best medical therapy as he was sent home without being provided with his aspirin, clopidogrel or high-dose statin therapy. He also has fairly restricted neck movements, with the patient saying that he has had issues with his neck for decades. You can also see a small horizontal scan in the region of his thyroid – the patient says that he had his thyroid removed a few years back and he is on thyroid replacement. The patient has also not had his full blood count checked in over 3 years, and he does not have a valid ECG. What would you do now?

A   Just get on with the operation. You have a busy theatre list and a fem-distal bypass to do after this carotid endarterectomy. If you spend another hour or so trying to get this carotid sorted your theatre list may run out of time to do the second case.

B   Don't proceed with this carotid endarterectomy. You have been duped. If you do proceed there would be a fairly high chance things may backfire on you, and it will be you who gets the blame if things go wrong.

C   Get the patient to down some aspirin, clopidogrel and statin tablets. Pressure the nursing staff to do an urgent ECG. Pressure the foundation doctor to get some up-to-date bloods. Pester the ENT core trainee to do a quick indirect larynoscopy. Do some rapid chiropractic adjustment of this patient's neck to improve his range of neck movement. This can all be achieved in around 1 hour. If all sorted in a timely fashion then proceed with the intended operation.

D   Get a second opinion from a consultant colleague, with the high likelihood that you will not proceed today. If the relevant work-up in completed and things seem favourable, to consider re-listing in a few days time.

✓ E   Have an honest conversation with the patient and explain that you do not think he has been worked up suitably to enable you to proceed safely with the intended operation today. Apologise to him. Arrange for a suitable reassessment/reappraisal of his options in a timely manner.

If the patient had been suitable for a carotid endarterectomy, what would be your chosen approach?

A   Excision of a diseased segment and interposition repair using reversed GSV.

B   Eversion endarterectomy.

C   Bovine or Dacron patch repair.

D   Cervical vein patch repair.

✓ E   Dealer's choice I guess … but I haven't heard of option A being used before, and that usually means it is the wrong answer.

You decide to do a bovine patch repair under general anaesthetic using a shunt. You use clips to close the skin. The operation seems to have gone well and you see the patient in recovery 10 minutes post-op. The patient seems to be moving all four limbs and indeed he is writhing around in bed. You go back to theatre to get ready for your next fem-distal bypass. Two minutes later, your anaesthetist runs into theatre and asks you to come straight back to recovery again. He says that the patient has a large neck haematoma. You go to see the patient in recovery and there is a very large haematoma in the neck that is expanding in front of you. What would your management plan be now?

   A Rush the patient straight back into theatre.

   B Remove the skin clips in recovery to decompress the haematoma (*this is likely to just be a venous ooze*).

✓ C Speak to the anaesthetist and highlight that the current priority is to secure the airway (*i.e. the focus should be on intubating the patient as soon as possible*).

   D Apply very firm pressure over the neck haematoma (*pressing down hard enough to stop any further haematoma expansion*).

   E Send the patient for an urgent CT angiogram.

The patient is intubated and taken back to theatre within a few minutes. Upon removing the skin clips, you are immediately met with fresh red blood that is seeping outwards from within the platysma closure layer. Once the platysma is opened, there is profuse active arterial bleeding coming from the inferior aspect of the bovine patch that has dehisced over a distance of around 1 cm (*and the carotid artery wall seems to have similarly torn at this area also*). What is your immediate management plan?

   A Suture repair of bleeding points using 4-0 Prolene.

   B Proximal and distal control, then suture repair using 5-0 or 6-0 Prolene.

   C Proximal and distal control, then take patch off, then re-shunt, then re-do the patch repair.

✓ D Proximal and distal control, then take patch off, then re-shunt, then re-do patch repair, then leave drain in neck, washout of neck using 2 litres of warm normal saline, and 48 hours of IV antibiotics post-op.

   E Proximal and distal control, then suture repair using 3-0 Prolene, washout of neck using 1 litre of warm normal saline, then leave drain in neck, standard antibiotic prophylaxis.

The patient has a re-do patch repair with shunting, and a 14-French drain is left in situ. This re-do operation was performed under general anaesthesia. The patient wakes up in recovery and you are called to see him because he is now not moving his right arm or right leg, and he has speech disturbance and a facial droop. He is moving his left arm and left leg normally. What are you going to do now?

   A Rush the patient back to theatre again for a further patch thrombectomy (*accepting that you are really now in a bad place but the most likely diagnosis is that the patch has thrombosed*).

   B Urgent CTA carotidsand intra-cranial circulation

   C Conservative management.

✓ D Urgent CTA carotids and intra-cranial circulation and CT brain (+/– *take back to theatre for patch thrombectomy or possibly urgent referral to neurointerventionl radiology for suction thrombectomy etc.*).

   E Urgent thrombolysis.

CASE REFLECTIONS

This initially was a real case *but as the case progressed the complications were fabricated. The real-life case itself had zero complications.* Indeed, the complications described here are simply an "orgy" of the complications we all worry about around the time of carotid surgery, and those that have educational value to discuss. I am just going to list some learning points and areas for reflection:

- All patients being considered for carotid intervention should be on best medical therapy. In my book (*literally*) this means aspirin, clopidogrel and high-dose statin. If a patient cannot or will not go on best medical therapy, I would consider this a ***BIG RED FLAG***. Indeed, I was referred a patient a few months ago for consideration of a carotid endarterectomy ... but the patient said that he did not agree with statin therapy because the evidence for it was weak, aspirin and clopidogrel he also did not agree with because they carried bleeding risks and the evidence for them was weak, and that he believed in healthy eating and herbal remedies, etc. ... suffice to say, he did ***not*** get a carotid endarterectomy.

- Remember that the "difficult" carotid endarterectomies are largely predictable pre-operatively. Watch out for patients with short thick necks that have a limited range of movement. Also use the dual imaging to get an idea of how high the ICA lesion is. For example, if you can see the distal ICA on the carotid duplex, this largely means that it cannot be a high lesion. If the MRA/CTA suggests the lesion is below the angle of the mandible this again suggests it is not a high lesion. Personally, I prefer CTA to MRA. I find that it easier to confirm how high the lesion is on CTA, and get a better idea of the nature of ICA disease on CTA. This is personal preference of course.

- Watch out for previous surgery in the neck. This should alert you to the possibility of a previous asymptomatic cranial nerve injury (*i.e. recurrent laryngeal/hypoglossal*). If you are considering carotid endarterectomy I would recommend asking ENT to do an indirect laryngoscopy. If you accidently cause a cranial nerve injury and the patient already has one on the other side, both vocal cords may end up being collapsed and the patient is going to need an emergency tracheostomy. Prevention is better than cure here.

- If a patient has a haematoma in the neck in theatre recovery or on the ward, then it is likely going to be due to a small venous ooze in the superficial layers. However, within the specific context of carotid surgery, if you have concluded that the patient needs to be returned to theatre I would recommend ***ASSUMING THE WORST***, i.e. that the patch or suture-line is potentially compromised. ***This does not mean that the patch or suture-line is compromised*** – it is simply a defence mechanism in case you do feel tempted to start removing sutures or clips in theatre recovery. I am not directly or indirectly aware of a specific case, but over the years I have heard various "stories" (*which now probably fit within the realm of folklore*) of junior vascular surgeons removing skin clips from the neck of post-op carotid endarterectomy patients to decompress a neck haematoma because of concerns about airway compromise. In these stories, the neck suddenly "blows" in recovery with catastrophic haemorrhage ensuing. What I was taught (*by my mentors*) is that if you have a concern about a neck haematoma in theatre recovery or on the ward, the ***first priority is the airway***. This means you deliberately have a conversation with a senior anaesthetist (*i.e. a consultant*) and get the patient intubated sooner rather than later. Once this is sorted, then you get the patient back to theatre to start opening up the neck wound and dealing with any mischief related to bleeding. ***The place to be "messing around" with neck wounds after a carotid endarterectomy is in theatre,*** not *in theatre recovery or on the ward*.

- If a patch has exploded in recovery and there is a big hole in your repair and a torn arterial wall … I would just re-shunt the patient and do the patch again. If it is a single tiny bleeding point then pragmatically a quick suture repair seems reasonable on the other hand. You have to be pragmatic here and make sensible decisions that reflect the clinical context.

- The final complication you witnessed in this case is the patient who has had a stroke and you see the result in theatre recovery. It is always much more painful when the patient is waking up from a general anaesthetic because you do not know if the patient is not moving their legs or arms because the anaesthetic has not worn off (*and you should keep your fingers crossed and wait a bit longer*) or does the patient actually have genuine neurological signs? The causes of stroke in this context include patch thrombosis, distal embolisation or an intra-cranial haemorrhage or possibly cerebral hyper-perfusion and oedema. I am not going to go into the specific management plans for each of these as they are available in other texts. However, the point I am trying to make in this case is that these sorts of complications need to be carefully considered *before* you commit to a carotid endarterectomy. If you have a patient who has a short thick neck, a terrible range of neck movement, scars in his neck from previous surgery, a high lesion on CTA/MRA/duplex, is not compliant with best medical therapy, has polycythaemia … then you are asking for trouble. Therefore if you turn up on the day of surgery and are confronted with a patient like this then I would recommend taking some big steps back and asking yourself if the risks of carotid endarterectomy truly outweigh the benefits. With the final picture of the patient waking up in theatre with what is clearly a dense hemiplegia, the management approach is controversial. Some may argue that this clinical picture within the hyperacute setting should mandate an immediate return to theatre for what is likely a carotid patch thrombosis, and this answer is not necessarily incorrect. However, in our specific case, things are not so straightforward. The patient could have a dissected ICA secondary to panicked shunting at the time of the return to theatre for bleeding. The patient may already have embolised into his MCA during the previous take-back (i.e. intra-operative stroke), and if you take him back to theatre again now you are then condemned to re-open the patch for a second time, and this may not be necessary. Indeed, a CTA may instead show clot in the MCA and neuro-interventional radiology may be able to suck the clot out. Within this specific context of our patient waking up with right-sided hemiplegia after already being taken back to theatre once before for bleeding … I would be inclined to get a rapid CT angiogram of the extra- and intra-cranial vessels as well as a CT brain. If the patch has thrombosed then I guess another trip to theatre may be justified … although another trip back to theatre is generally not a "good look" and the case is now basically becoming a disaster … the overall outlook would appear pretty bleak at this junction whatever you decide to do. The main learning point here is that ***prevention is better than cure***.

- Indeed, the final message from this case is to make sure you are taking decent bites of the patch and carotid wall when you are doing your patch repair, ***and*** spend around 5–10 minutes at the end of your case truly achieving haemostasis in the neck. There is no point rushing these cases. If you rush these cases, all that happens is you end up spending much longer seeing the patient in recovery, applying pressure dressings to the neck, deliberating on whether or not to take the patient back to theatre, etc.

A 72-year-old male is visiting the United Kingdom to celebrate a close family member's birthday. This patient used to live in the UK but decided to move abroad around 4 years ago. He has presented to an A&E department 25 minutes away from your tertiary vascular centre. He is complaining of severe abdominal pain for the past few days (*that which has been steadily worsening over the past 3 months*). He is reported to be haemodynamically stable. His past medical history includes: previous EVAR performed in the same hospital 7 years ago, atrial fibrillation on warfarin, hypercholesterolaemia, hypertension, mild chronic kidney disease (eGFR 58), and right leg embolectomy and calf fasciotomies 7 years ago (*performed around 3 months after his original EVAR*). He is otherwise independent with an exercise tolerance of 1 mile (*and no significant cardiorespiratory pathology*).

What is your working diagnosis (*having not seen the patient yet or reviewed any current or previous imaging*)?

✓ A Symptomatic AAA sac.
  B Ruptured AAA sac.
  C Pancreatitis.
  D Perforated gastric ulcer.
  E Thoracic aortic dissection.

You receive a very brief update about this patient by your own vascular registrar. They have been phoned directly by the A&E middle grade in the referring hospital. The concern is that he has a symptomatic AAA – they have done a CT angiogram which apparently shows a large AAA sac and "worrying signs." This hospital used to have a vascular surgery department, but it no longer does due to centralisation of vascular services. How would you respond to this?

  A Ask your junior to get back in contact with the A&E team and instruct them to do a more thorough work-up before assuming this is a vascular surgery problem.
  B Take the details of the patient from your junior and start to do some investigating yourself.
  C Bury your head in the sand and hope that the matter just goes away – this is not a problem for the parent hospital to deal with.
  D Instruct your junior to inform the parent A&E team to get the general surgery team in the parent hospital to assess the patient first, and then get the general surgeons to contact you back directly if they truly think this is a vascular surgery problem.
✓ E Take sufficient information from your vascular junior about the clinical problem, the patient details, exactly where the patient is, review the medical notes and imaging yourself, and then plan to get back in contact with the referring A&E team as necessary.

Your registrar reads the CT angiogram report to you:

> *Infra-renal aortic sac measures 95 × 101 mm. The main body of the EVAR is free floating. The right EVAR limb lies on the edge of the aneurysm in the very proximal CIA. The left limb has maintained a seal zone. No obvious endoleak detected. There is no evidence of AAA sac rupture, but on the right and proximal aspect of the sac wall there is minimal fluid seen, and this is suspicioun for imminent rupture.*

The CTA images that correspond to this report are seen in Figure 13.1.

DOI: 10.1201/9781003497042-13

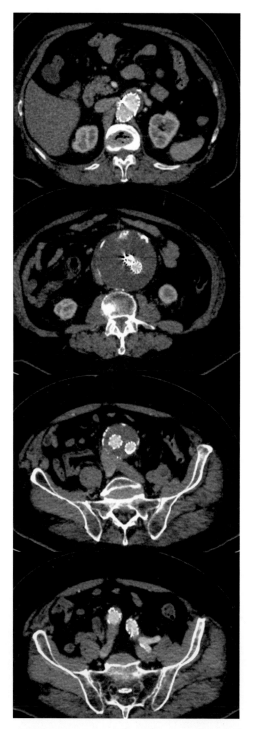

Figure 13.1 CTA when patient presents acutely with worsening abdominal pain in neighbouring A&E.

What are your thoughts at this stage?

   A Patient requires at the very least a complex endovascular solution and I work in the central/tertiary aortic centre. Therefore, I accept the patient for immediate blue light transfer.

✓ B Patient may require a complex endovascular solution or emergency explantation. I work in the central/tertiary aortic centre. Therefore, I will accept the patient for immediate blue light transfer.

   C I need a few hours to review all the imaging and only if I think there is a viable endovascular or open surgical solution will I then accept the patient for transfer.

   D The patient can go home, but then come back to the vascular surgery assessment unit the following day for assessment.

   E This patient can be discharged home and come back to the aortic clinic next week with a plan for urgent outpatient work-up.

You telephone your vascular interventional radiology consultant colleague on-call and ask them to review the imaging. The vascular radiology opinion is that there is no explicit endoleak, but the top end seal zone looks compromised and although they could extend the right limb of the EVAR, it is better for the patient to be in the main aortic centre as there is a high likelihood that the top end will also need sorting (*would need axillary cut-down and branch repair with extension of right iliac limb*). This could possibly be a type 5 endoleak, i.e. increase in aneurysm sac without identifiable endoleak. The alternative is a type 4 endoleak due to graft porosity. There are signs of impending rupture.

Unsurprisingly you accept the patient for blue light transfer to your centre. The patient appears 25 minutes later and the patient is in A&E majors. The patient appears stable but is in a lot of pain (*diffuse abdominal pain, but specifically most tender in right iliac fossa*). He is obese (*BMI 35*). He does seem to be showing signs of peritoneal irritation. A healthcare assistant hands you a venous blood gas result (Figure 13.2). What do you make of it?

   A Patient is acidotic with a raised lactate, but haemoglobin is normal. Given right sided pain this is likely to be acute perforated appendicitis. Patient needs an urgent general surgery review.

   B Patient has diffuse abdominal pain with signs of peritoneal irritation. Therefore acute mesenteric ischaemia is the most likely diagnosis (*i.e. SMA embolic/thrombotic occlusion*).

   C Patient has a symptomatic AAA and is simply dehydrated. He requires IV fluids and analgesia, admission to the high dependency unit for close observation overnight, and aortic MDT discussion the following morning.

✓ D The patient has a massive AAA with signs of impending rupture. If it looks like a duck, swims like a duck, and quacks like a duck, then it probably is a duck, i.e. his AAA has likely ruptured. The A&E consultant needs to be updated, the patient needs moving to resus, and he needs an urgent repeat CT angiogram.

   E Clinically it could very well be a ruptured AAA. However, his haemoglobin is normal on the blood gas, and there is simply no way your night shift on-call could be this unlucky.

Please review the CTA (Figure 13.3) – what is your working diagnosis now?

   A Type 2 endoleak with AAA sac rupture.

✓ B Type 1b endoleak with AAA sac rupture.

   C Type 1a endoleak with AAA sac rupture.

   D Type 3 endoleak with AAA sac rupture.

   E Type 1b endoleak without AAA sac rupture.

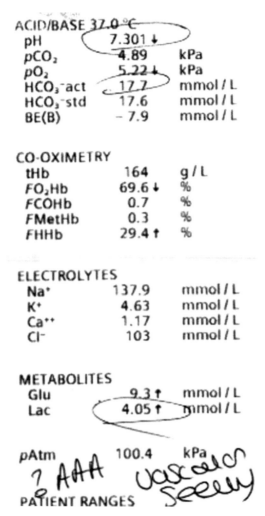

ACID/BASE 37.0 °C
pH	7.301 ↓	
pCO$_2$	4.89	kPa
pO$_2$	5.22 ↓	kPa
HCO$_3^-$ act	17.7	mmol / L
HCO$_3^-$ std	17.6	mmol / L
BE(B)	− 7.9	mmol / L

CO-OXIMETRY
tHb	164	g / L
FO$_2$Hb	69.6 ↓	%
FCOHb	0.7	%
FMetHb	0.3	%
FHHb	29.4 ↑	%

ELECTROLYTES
Na$^+$	137.9	mmol / L
K$^+$	4.63	mmol / L
Ca^{++}	1.17	mmol / L
Cl$^-$	103	mmol / L

METABOLITES
Glu	9.3 ↑	mmol / L
Lac	4.05 ↑	mmol / L

pAtm   100.4   kPa

? AAA   vascular

PATIENT RANGES

Figure 13.2   Venous blood gas result upon arrival in your A&E department.

What would be your immediate management plan?

A NBM, activate major transfusion protocol, seek urgent haematology advice and reverse warfarin, take immediately to theatre for EVAR explantation and bifurcated graft repair.

B NBM, activate major transfusion protocol, seek urgent haematology advice and reverse warfarin, take immediately to IR theatre for right iliac limb extension.

C NBM, activate major transfusion protocol, seek urgent haematology advice and reverse warfarin, take immediately to theatre to IR theatre for right iliac limb extension, axillary cutdown and branch repair of visceral segment.

✓ D NBM, activate major transfusion protocol, seek urgent haematology advice and reverse warfarin, call for help from senior and experienced vascular consultant surgeon and seek further vascular radiology opinion on viability of endovascular options available with context of rupture and now visible type 1b endoleak from right limb of EVAR.

E Palliate the patient.

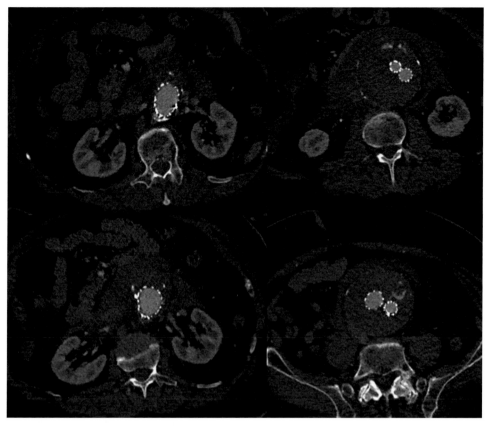

Figure 13.3 Repeat CTA in light of peritoneal irritation, acidosis, and raised lactate on venous blood gas.

WHAT ACTUALLY HAPPENED AT THIS POINT?

Please see Figure 13.4 for the final decision-making process.

What would be your surgical approach to explanting this EVAR and then doing an open AAA repair?

A Full explantation, i.e. supra-coeliac control first and then pull entirety of graft out.

✓ B Partial explantation, i.e. use some sternal wire cutters and divide EVAR in the infra-renal segment and then suture in a new graft to this remaining proximal EVAR device and infra-renal aortic neck.

C Full explantation without supra-coeliac control. Just grab the EVAR and rip it downwards and then be prepared to apply an infra-renal clamp immediately afterwards once it is out.

D Do not explant the EVAR at all. Just try to get a big tie around the infra-renal neck to snug it down onto the EVAR in case there is a type 1a endoleak, and then do something similar for the right iliac limb (*or suture the right iliac limb to the native common iliac artery to secure it in place*).

E Accepting that there is likely just a type 1B endoleak secondary to a free-floating right iliac limb, just ligate the right iliac limb and then do a femoral-femoral crossover (left to right).

Ruptured AAA

Patient acidotic and now tachycardic

New endoleak around right limb

Mini-MDT with

Extending right limb of EVAR could be considered as damage control procedure, however this does nothing to sort out the top end and patient could continue to ooze from rupture site (working diagnosis was that this may have been due to endotension originally)

Consensus opinion supported open repair, although you could argue the case either way

Caught between rock and a hard place, could do full open repair with high risk of death but this is the definitive repair option and he sounds fit enough for this, or right iliac limb extension as damage control procedure and maybe FEVAR at a later date (would need to do right groin cutdown anyways as his groins are so deep!)

I think patient is fit enough for open and this is what I think is the best option

Dr   , Dr   and Mr   think open repair is justifiable and agree with plan for open

I spoke to patient and said I thought open repair was better option for him

Very high chance of death (I said > 80% chance of him not surviving)

Patient trusts our judgement and is happy to proceed with open repair

I advised him to speak to his family and say his goodbyes

Consent form completed

Safe surgery checklist completed

Massive transfusion protocol activated

Optiplex and vitamin K being given

Mr   came to see patient in HOT resus and agrees with plan for open repair tonight

Figure 13.4 Final surgical plan.

What do you make of the image and report from his original EVAR 7 years ago (Figure 13.5)? Would it influence your decision-making around full explantation vs partial explantation?

A   Just looks like a standard infra-renal EVAR to me. EVAR will likely come out easily.

B   Clearly at the time of the original EVAR there were issues with a type 1a endoleak. There is a cuff extension there. Henceforth, if I start yanking on that with no discretion I could easily tear the visceral segment and then it is game over. However … I really don't have any other option here. If the patient needs an explant, then I must explant everything. Game on.

✓ C   Perhaps given the fact that there is extra metalwork at the top end I should consider trying to pursue a damage control approach, i.e. keep things simple and focus on getting the patient out of trouble. If I can get away with a partial explant this is probably a more pragmatic approach.

D   This patient is obese and getting supra-coeliac control is going to be difficult. Removing all of the EVAR is going to be risky and dangerous and therefore not a viable option. I think therefore the only option here is palliation.

E   I can explant everything. If the visceral segment tears then I guess I will have to do a supra-coeliac-SMA/renal/renal bypass. No big deal.

The operative images are visible in Figure 13.6.

CASE REFLECTIONS

This was an absolute beast of a case. It has been suitably amended so the case remains anonymous, but for all intents and purposes, the overall learning points are genuine. I was on call for 24 hours, and it was Sunday evening. I had spent the entire day in the hospital not doing anything exciting and thought it was the perfect time to go home as nothing was happening. I had literally left the building when my registrar phoned to update me about a phone call he had received from a neighbouring A&E department. This patient was being sold to us as a symptomatic AAA. I did a fairly thorough remote review of whatever case notes were available, reviewed the previous imaging, spoke to various colleagues in my department, and to A&E in both this referring unit and my own A&E department. To cut a long story short, the patient was blue-lighted across very quickly.

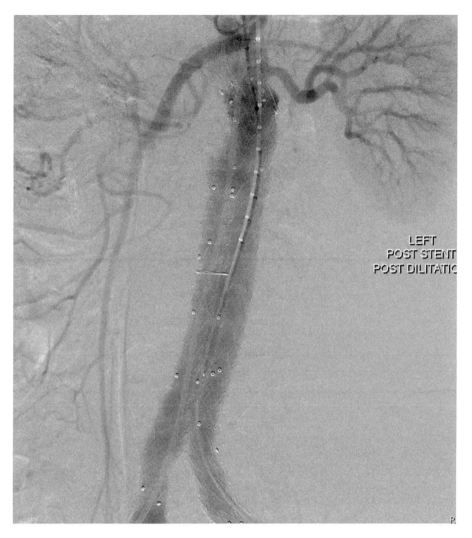

LEFT
POST STENT
POST DILITATIC

STENT GRAFT ABDOMINAL AORTA :

Body of the graft placed from the left side. One extension on the left side and 2 extensions on the right side.

Moulding balloon used junctions. Angiogram showed type I endoleak. The body of the graft was moulded. There was still some evidence of type I endo leak.

Hence a cuff was used

Following this angiogram showed good result and there is no evidence of any endo leak. Satisfactory position of the graft. Groin closure by surgeons.

Figure 13.5 Original EVAR pertinent information.

When the patient arrived I was expecting just to say hello and then set him up for a discussion in the aortic MDT the following morning. However, it quickly became apparent that he had ruptured his AAA (*likely during the ambulance transit to my unit*). At that point decision-making became relatively simple, mainly because I had already had all the relevant conversations about possible plans before the patient had arrived. Indeed, there was already a plan in place that if the patient ruptured he was heading for explantation, i.e. open AAA repair. There was some

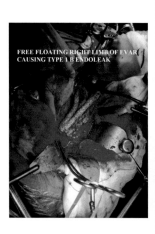
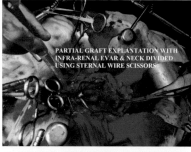
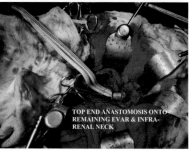
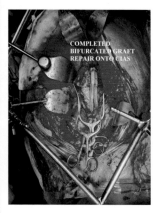

Figure 13.6 Operative images.

controversy about whether we should just reline his right iliac limb as a quick bailout solution. There was further controversy about whether the top end seal zone was also compromised. Time was limited here … but the final decision was to commit to explantation and AAA repair. Essentially, I thought that a straightforward endovascular solution was wishful thinking, and in my eyes this patient was either for explantation and open AAA repair or palliation. The patient (*unsurprisingly*) did not want to die, and this made the decision-making easy. I simply called a senior consultant vascular surgeon to come and assist me and we proceeded to partial explantation. We already had planned to do a partial explantation using some cardiac sternal wire cutters as opposed to a full explantation because getting supra-coeliac control in such a large abdomen would have been very difficult, and the extra cuff extension meant trying to pull it all out would be more difficult.

In the end, the patient sailed through the operation and went home one week later. Clinic follow-up 6 weeks later found him to be doing very well apart from some minor liver function test derangement (*likely as a result of some ischaemic damage from the AAA rupture*).

CORE LESSONS
- Take endoleaks and expanding AAA sacs seriously.
- EVAR may be minimally invasive, but there are long-term risks which can be catastrophic. If a patient is fit for open AAA repair, this may be their best option from the outset.
- If you are considering an EVAR in a patient, be very wary if they have plans to live abroad in the future. This is a very easy way for a patient to get lost to follow-up. Essentially, surveillance of EVAR patients is of crucial importance … and needs to be taken into account before you commit to an EVAR. Be particularly careful of patients visiting your country from abroad who then present with a symptomatic AAA … if you put an EVAR in make sure that the patient is aware of the importance of surveillance when they go back home.

- If you are dealing with "big problems" like this, then don't deal with it on your own. Call for help, and preferably call someone who is a lot more experienced than you and has grey hair (*actually I have noticed that my hair is getting greyer these days*).

- When dealing with complex catastrophic vascular problems be realistic and pragmatic. In this case there were various surgical and endovascular options being suggested and considered … but I was the consultant on the ground when all this kicked off, and I had limited time to think. In the end I believed partial explantation and open AAA repair with a bifurcated graft was this patient's best option, and I still do – *and not just because the patient did well*. I suspect if we had tried to reline his right iliac EVAR limb the wire would have been floating around in his massive AAA sac for an hour, and then we would have been forced to open him up anyways when he had lost a further 3 litres of blood into his retroperitoneum. Ultimately, vascular surgery is about making decisions, and decisions carry both risks and benefits. With cases like this however you cannot really sit on the fence, you just have to weigh up the options and then *make a decision in a timely fashion*. Whatever decision you make anticipate that somebody else may well have made a different decision if they were presented with the exact same situation – *each to their own*.

- The final lesson is this – if you strongly suspect a big problem is coming your way, then use the time before the patient arrives to review the notes and images, discuss with colleagues, and start planning what you might do if the worst-case scenario materialises. At least then if you do encounter the worst-case scenario later, your thinking process has already taken place and you will be ready to start executing your plan at a moment's notice. In this case, I had already decided that if the patient ruptured his AAA I was going to open him up and explant the EVAR. As such, I had already phoned a senior consultant colleague and fired this warning shot 45 minutes prior to the patient arriving. Essentially, I did not "phone a friend" primarily to ask a question about management, but instead primarily to recruit his assistance if the patient did rupture and I did intend to proceed with explantation and open repair. When his CTA did confirm AAA rupture, I literally picked up my mobile phone and phoned my senior colleague and simply said: "He has ruptured." My colleague already knew what the plan was and was already poised to come and join me in theatre. Essentially, this is something of a traffic light system. If you are already poised at **AMBER** then you can very quickly transition to **GREEN**. However, if your baseline is **RED**, you then have to transition to **AMBER** and then to **GREEN** before you can start moving (*which involves more time spent thinking, deliberating, conversing, seeking others' opinions … and more time for the patient to bleed and go into multi-organ failure*). Basically, if you have a massive case coming your way, you should ideally be positioned at **AMBER** before you even see the patient.

A 39-year-old male is referred to you via telephone from a GP. This patient has presented with left hand "pins and needles" and absent wrist pulses. His symptoms started suddenly 1 month ago. He went to see his GP today because his symptoms have not resolved and the patient is worried there is something sinister wrong. What is your first impression?

   A This patient has a threatened limb and requires urgent revascularisation. He needs to be seen now and rushed to the operating theatre.

   B This is likely a delayed presentation of acute limb ischaemia, most likely Rutherford 1 ischaemia. I am not going to rush into anything crazy here, but I will see the patient.

   C This patient likely has carpal tunnel syndrome and the GP probably does not know how to feel a pulse. I am going to reject this referral and advise the GP to refer the patient for nerve conduction studies.

   D This patient likely has cervical nerve root compression. He requires an MRI and referral to a spinal surgeon.

✓ E GP says there are no wrist pulses and the patient has symptoms suggesting neurological compromise. I am not going to make any premature assumptions. I will see the patient urgently to be on the safe side.

The patient arrives in the surgical assessment area 1.5 hours later. He looks well. He greets you and is clearly not in significant pain. His right and left upper limb movements appear grossly normal. His left hand does look pale compared to the right. The power in the left upper limb is 5/5. The sensation is intact, although there are reports of minor "pins and needles" that have not deteriorated further over the past month. The capillary refill time in the left hand is 3 seconds. There is no tissue loss, ulceration, or gangrene. You can feel a proximal subclavian artery pulse, but nil distally. What is your working diagnosis?

   A Delayed presentation of acute embolic upper limb ischaemia – Rutherford 2A.

✓ B Delayed presentation of acute embolic upper limb ischaemia – Rutherford 1.

   C Chronic limb-threatening ischaemia of the upper limb.

   D Likely previous aortic dissection and left subclavian artery origin compromise.

   E Likely delayed presentation of upper limb DVT (*which is making pulse assessment challenging*).

The patient informs you that his left arm symptoms suddenly developed when he was out walking. He says that he was carrying his dog in his left arm. There are no significant medical problems. He is not a smoker. There is no foreign travel/illicit substance abuse/fevers, sweats, or shakes. There are no chest or back pain or palpitations reported. There are no reports of amaurosis fugax or anything resembling a stroke or mini-stroke. There is a family history of heart valve issues. The patient has normal right arm and lower limb pulses (*all regular*). On auscultation of the chest, the heart sounds are normal (*no obvious murmurs*). What is your primary differential diagnosis at this point?

   A Cardioembolic ischaemia.

   B Thrombotic ischaemia due to underlying upper limb atherosclerotic disease.

   C Lower limb DVT with right-to-left atrial shunt and secondary embolic upper limb ischaemia.

   D Cervical rib pathology.

✓ E Could be anything to be perfectly honest. Patient needs a thorough work-up.

DOI: 10.1201/9781003497042-14

What would your work-up be?

  A ECG +/− ambulatory ECG, echocardiogram and left arm arterial duplex.

✓ B ECG +/− ambulatory ECG, echocardiogram, thoracic outlet x-ray to rule out cervical ribs, CT arch of aorta and left upper limb, bloods (FBC, U&Es, LFTs, clotting, TFTs, HBA1c, lipid screen, calcium, magnesium, vasculitic screen, thrombosis screen, CRP)

  C Urgent outpatient MRA left arm and arch of aorta, ambulatory ECG, and echocardiogram.

  D Urgent CT angiogram of the arch of aorta alone.

  E Left arm arterial duplex alone.

What do you make of the x-ray (Figure 14.1)?

  A Normal.

✓ B Bilateral cervical ribs.

  C Left cervical rib.

  D Right cervical rib.

  E Pancoast tumour on the left.

What do you make of the CT angiogram (Figure 14.2)?

  A Acute embolic occlusion of the subclavian artery.

  B In situ thrombosis of the diseased subclavian artery.

✓ C Likely thrombosed subclavian artery aneurysm.

  D Dissected left subclavian artery.

  E Malignant growth that has invaded the subclavian artery.

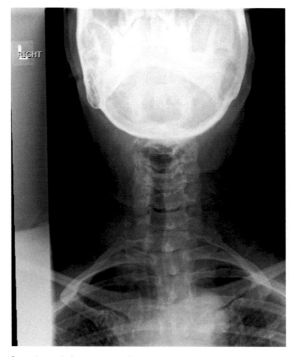

Figure 14.1 X-ray of neck and thoracic outlet.

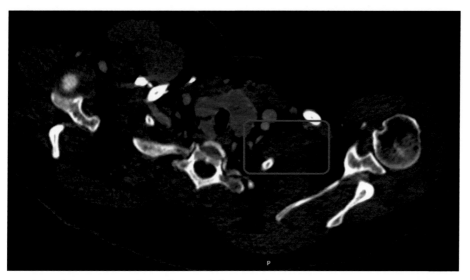

Figure 14.2   CT angiogram for ischaemic left upper limb.

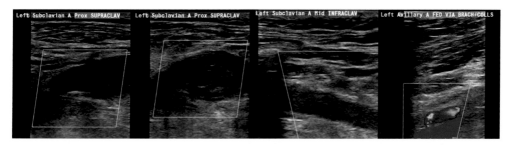

Figure 14.3   Left arm arterial duplex.

The patient has a subsequent arterial duplex to visualise the subclavian artery. What do you make of the images (Figure 14.3) and this report:

Thrombosed supraclavicular subclavian artery aneurysm with a maximum diameter of 1.7 cm in LS and 1.6 cm in TS. No flow is seen within the infra-clavicular subclavian artery. Flow reconstitutes in the axillary artery via branch vessels/collaterals. Non-occlusive thrombus can be seen within the proximal brachial artery. The mid-brachial artery is patent, monophasic flow of 23 cm/sec. Thrombus can be seen within the distal brachial artery where a large collateral vessel is demonstrated, the thrombus extends into the proximal ulnar artery for 2.3 cm caudal to the bifurcation. Monophasic flow seen throughout the remainder of the ulnar artery. The radial artery demonstrates monophasic flow, but flow occludes cranial to the wrist and cannot been seen into the hand.

In light of the clinical and radiological findings, what is your impression and management plan at this stage?

   A Acutely thrombosed left subclavian artery aneurysm with distal embolisation. Patient requires an urgent brachial embolectomy.

✓ B Delayed presentation of a thrombosed left subclavian artery aneurysm with distal embolisation. Patient has a viable hand. Manage conservatively with anticoagulation (*risks of revascularisation outweigh the benefits*).

C Delayed presentation of a thrombosed left subclavian artery aneurysm with distal embolisation. Patient has a viable hand but some "pins and needles" that have been present for a month. Patient requires urgent cervical rib resection, proximal subclavian to distal axillary interposition graft repair.

D Delayed presentation of a thrombosed left subclavian artery aneurysm with distal embolisation. Patient has a viable hand but some "pins and needles" that have been present for a month. Patient requires urgent cervical rib resection, proximal subclavian to distal axillary interposition graft repair +/− brachial artery embolectomy/jump grafting onto distal brachial artery.

E Delayed presentation of a thrombosed left subclavian artery aneurysm with distal embolisation. Patient has a viable hand but some "pins and needles" that have been present for a month. Patient requires thrombolysis to clear the run-off and then subclavian artery aneurysm repair.

The patient is counselled on the options available. A joint decision is made to manage the left arm conservatively. The patient asks if you if intervention might be required for the right cervical rib. His right arm is currently completely asymptomatic and he has a full complement of right arm pulses. The right arm is the dominant arm. What would be your response?

A Let's forget about it and not go looking for problems.

✓ B You will review his imaging in the vascular MDT. If there is radiological evidence of damage to the right subclavian artery and/or evidence of impingement, there might be an argument in support of prophylactic cervical rib resection.

C Plan for a repeat CT angiogram of her right arm in 5 years.

D Plan for a repeat MR angiogram of her right arm in 10 years.

E Plan for a repeat arterial duplex of her right arm in 3 years.

What do you make of these CTA and duplex images (Figure 14.4) along with this duplex report:

Normal calibre supraclavicular subclavian artery with a maximum diameter of 0.83 cm. Multiphasic flow throughout the subclavian artery, triphasic flow throughout the axillary and brachial artery, and multiphasic flow throughout the radial and ulnar arteries to the level of the wrist. No thrombus, stenosis or aneurysm can be seen within the right upper limb. At rest the mid-infra-clavicular subclavian artery demonstrates multiphasic flow. Upon raising the arm, flow ranges from no flow, dampened monophasic flow of 10 cm/sec to increased velocity monophasic disturbed flow, PSV = 248 cm/sec (positional with arm movement). In Roos provocation flow is disturbed and monophasic, PSV = 243 cm/sec. Hyperaemic flow is noted post Roos provocation

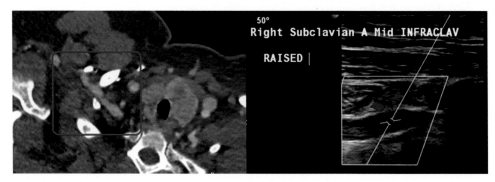

Figure 14.4   CT angiogram and right arm arterial duplex.

returning to multiphasic within seconds. Impingement on B-mode can be seen within the artery at the site of the clavicle.

A There is evidence of minor subclavian pinching on CTA with some post-stenotic dilatation. The duplex confirms that there is impingement around this exact area. However, the subclavian artery appears grossly normal on the CTA. The patient also remains asymptomatic. Therefore, the right cervical rib should be managed conservatively.

B There is evidence of minor subclavian pinching on CTA with some post-stenotic dilatation. The duplex confirms that there is impingement around this exact area. However, the patient remains asymptomatic, so to manage conservatively for the moment and repeat cross-sectional imaging in 3 years. If patient develops a subclavian artery aneurysm to surgical intervene at that stage.

C There is evidence of minor subclavian pinching on CTA with some post-stenotic dilatation. The duplex confirms that there is impingement around this exact area. However, the patient remains asymptomatic, so this should be managed conservatively.

D There is evidence of minor subclavian pinching on CTA with some post-stenotic dilatation. The duplex confirms that there is impingement around this exact area. The patient remains asymptomatic. However, there has already been a major ischaemic complication in the left arm (*which could have easily resulted in limb loss*), this is now his dominant arm, and there is already evidence of low level arterial damage to the right subclavian artery. If this is managed conservatively and then he develops the same problem in the right arm (*and loses the right arm*), it would be difficult to defend.

✓ E There is evidence of minor subclavian pinching on CTA with some post-stenotic dilatation. The duplex confirms that there is impingement around this exact area. The patient remains asymptomatic. However, there has already been a major ischaemic complication in the left arm (*which could have easily resulted in limb loss*), this is now the dominant arm, and there is already evidence of low level arterial damage to the right subclavian artery. If this is managed conservatively and the patient subsequently develops the same problem in the right arm (*and loses the right arm*), it could be difficult to defend. However, exposing the patient to cervical rib resection also carries risks (*including iatrogenic injury to subclavian vein, artery, brachial plexus, pleura, and the phrenic nerve*). Such iatrogenic injuries could carry significant consequences also. Henceforth, I will counsel the patient on the options available for the right arm, highlight the risks and benefits, but I will still make a case to support prophylactic cervical rib resection. Ultimately it will be an informed patient decision.

Some images from the theatre are presented (Figures 14.5, 14.6, 14.7, and 14.8).

CASE REFLECTIONS

In this case the right cervical rib and first rib were resected to prevent further prophylactic damage to the right subclavian artery, and the left cervical rib was managed conservatively. Indeed, the left arm made significant improvements after being left well alone.

I think this case simply highlights the heart of surgery, i.e. weighing risks and benefits. This patient ironically went for surgery on the arm that was otherwise asymptomatic, and yet the arm that had a pretty bad vascular complication and was symptomatic did not get any surgery. Sounds counter-intuitive upon first impression. However, think of the parallel universe when this patient actually goes for the completely opposite management plan:

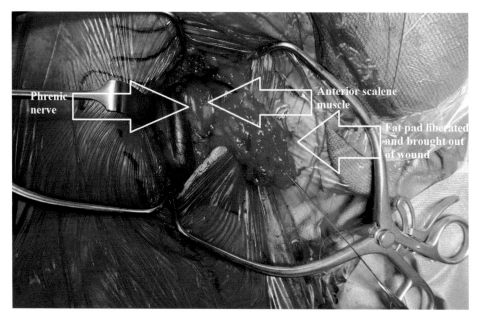

Figure 14.5 Right supraclavicular fat pad retraction.

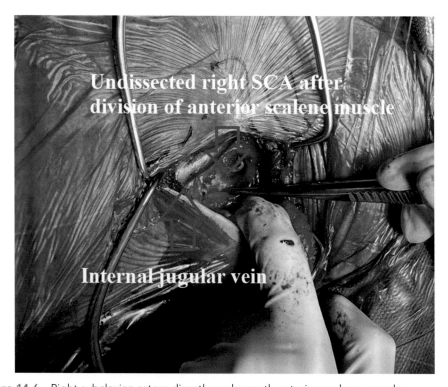

Figure 14.6 Right subclavian artery directly underneath anterior scalene muscle.

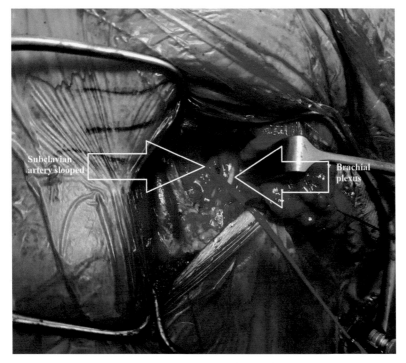

Figure 14.7   Right subclavian artery dissected and slooped to access cervical rib underneath.

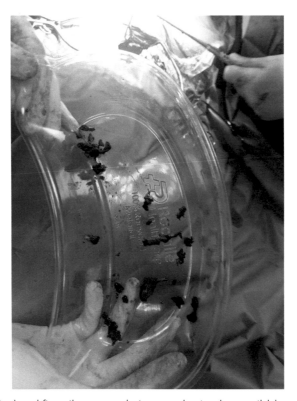

Figure 14.8   Cervical and first rib resected piecemeal using bone nibblers.

OPERATION NOTE

Left Cervical Rib and First Rib Resection with Left Subclavian Artery Aneurysm Repair (Subclavian to Axillary Artery Interposition Graft Using PTFE)

Complications:

1) Pneumothorax requiring chest drain insertion.

2) Early bypass occlusion (because the upper limb run-off is compromised).

3) Late bypass graft infection requiring explantation 6 months later.

4) Right upper limb ischaemia secondary to thrombosed right subclavian artery aneurysm 2 years later (*was managed conservatively with a plan for repeat right subclavian artery duplex in 3 years time*). This resulted in the patient losing the right arm above the elbow.

5) The patient remarks to you 4 years later (*when you are in court looking him in the eye*) that he was never fully informed about the risks related to the left arm surgery and in retrospect he never needed a bypass in the first place because his left arm was viable. He also then remarks that he was never told about the consequences of managing the right arm conservatively and that if he had known the same thing was likely to happen on the right as it did on the left he would have pushed harder for prophylactic right cervical rib resection and/or sought a second opinion, etc.

Essentially, when you are making surgical decisions you need to ask yourself what the likely predicted outcome is going to be. If you can honestly see yourself making a patient worse off by operating on them, then you probably should not operate on them. On the other hand, if you can honestly predict that the patient will deteriorate significantly if you manage them conservatively, then you probably should operate on them. Obviously, surgical decision-making is more complicated than this and there are many further nuances, but essentially this is what surgery is all about. The medicolegal element being introduced here is perhaps not of primary relevance to most readers of this book at this stage of their career. However, it is likely that at some point in your career you may find yourself facing complications that ultimately get escalated into the medicolegal realm. At this junction you may find yourself reading back through the medical notes to prepare your statement, and deeply regretting that you had not thoroughly documented that the patient was counselled on the options available including the risks and the benefits of each of the options. You may also find a scanned consent form with frankly illegible handwriting, and even you cannot decipher what was written within the risks section.

It is 11 pm and you are the vascular surgeon on-call. You are at home in bed sleeping when the phone rings. You answer the phone and it is an A&E core trainee from a hospital 20 minutes away. She asks if you are the on-call vascular surgeon, to which you answer yes. She says there is a 60-year-old man with an aortic dissection, and she has been asked by her consultant to refer to you. What are the first questions you should ask?

✓ A Have you seen the patient, and what type of aortic dissection is it (i.e. A or B)?
  B What is the patient's haemodynamic status?
  C What is the patient's lower limb pulse status?
  D When did the patient arrive and how long have the symptoms been going on for?
  E Has the patient had cross-sectional imaging?

The referring A&E doctor says that she has not seen the patient, and she does not know if it is a type A or type B dissection. She says that her consultant has seen the patient and she can read what he has documented in the medical notes. She can also read to you the CT angiogram report. How would you respond to this?

  A Tell her that she needs to get her consultant to call me.
✓ B Yes please read to me what your consultant has documented, and also what the CT report says.
  C Ask her to go and see the patient, take a full history and examination again, and then call me back in 20 minutes.
  D Tell her that she needs to first determine if this is a type A or type B dissection, and then only if it is a type B dissection is there any point continuing the conversation.
  E Tell her that she is telephoning a vascular surgery consultant at 11 pm and it is not ideal that she has not seen the patient, nor is it ideal that she does not know what type of aortic dissection it is.

The referring A&E doctor proceeds to give you a genuinely impressive description of what is going on with the patient (*she basically reads out what her consultant has documented in the notes*). This is the information you capture:

- 60-year-old man.
- Presented a few hours ago with severe sudden-onset interscapular pain and collapse.
- No past medical history of note, otherwise fit and well.
- No current medications.
- No drug allergies.
- Smoker of 15 cigarettes per day, minimal alcohol intake.
- Blood pressure now is 198/106 mmHg.
- Heart rate now is 88.
- No signs of stroke.
- Abdomen is soft and non-tender.
- Upper and lower limb pulses are normal, but the right leg pulses are weaker than the left.
- The patient is complaining of some minor pins and needles/numbness in the right foot, but the power and sensation are objectively intact.
- Blood results are: Hb 167, WBC 23, PLT 223, Na 141, K 3.9, urea 4.9, creatinine 87, clotting grossly normal.

DOI: 10.1201/9781003497042-15

- CT angiogram report:

There is a large mural thrombus which extends from the aortic arch down to the level of the iliac bifurcation and into the right external iliac artery. No corresponding hyperdensity is seen on the non-contrast study to suggest and intramural haematoma. A blush of contrast is seen extending from the aortic lumen into the thrombus approximately 5 cm downstream from the left subclavian artery in keeping with a penetrating atherosclerotic ulcer. A further possible ulcer is seen within the descending thoracic aorta. There is no intra-abdominal free fluid. Within the limitation of an arterial study, normal appearance of the visualised abdominal viscera. The visualised lungs are clear. No aggressive osseous lesion. Conclusion: Extensive mural thrombus as described above with a penetrating atherosclerotic ulcer in the descending thoracic aorta (and possibly a smaller penetrating ulcer distally). Urgent vascular referral recommended.

What would you say to the referring A&E clinician?

  A The report mentions that this is from the aortic arch downwards. Therefore, this is a problem for cardiac surgery. Please refer to them.

  B This sounds like a descending thoracic penetrating aortic ulcer +/− type B dissection with possible right acute lower limb ischaemia. I will review the imaging remotely from home and also liaise with my vascular radiology colleagues and get their opinion on the imaging. Can I take your contact details and call you back in a few minutes? If this genuinely is a type B dissection picture, I will take over the patient's care.

✓ C This sounds like a descending thoracic penetrating aortic ulcer +/− type B dissection with possible right acute lower limb ischaemia. I will review the imaging remotely from home and liaise with my vascular radiology colleagues for their opinion on the imaging. Can I take your contact details and call you back in a few minutes? If this genuinely is a type B dissection picture I will take over the patient's care. In the meantime, please can you insert an arterial line, commence the patient on intravenous beta-blockade, and aim for a systolic blood pressure $\leq$ 120 and a heart rate $\leq$ 60. Also, please keep the patient nil by mouth as I am concerned about the perfusion to the right leg.

  D All of these CT changes sound chronic to me. Please can you make sure the patient has had an ECG and a troponin checked as this could be a myocardial infarction.

  E Please can you refer this patient to your own intensive care unit for strict blood pressure control and a repeat CT angiogram in 48 hours time. If the CT shows worsening changes I will consider taking over this patient's care at that junction.

What do you make of the CT angiogram images which you are reviewing from home (Figure 15.1)?

✓ A Image quality isn't great, but looks like a type B dissection to me. I am also worried about the right iliac perfusion, although there does still seem to be contrast filling the right CFA. I am going to speak to vascular radiology and get their opinion on the imaging, but I am otherwise going to accept this patient under my care and arrange urgent transfer.

  B Type A dissection. Needs urgent referral to cardiac surgery.

  C Chronic changes only, nil concerning. Discharge from vascular surgery.

  D Left subclavian artery dissection.

  E Aortic arch dissection and large mediastinal haematoma.

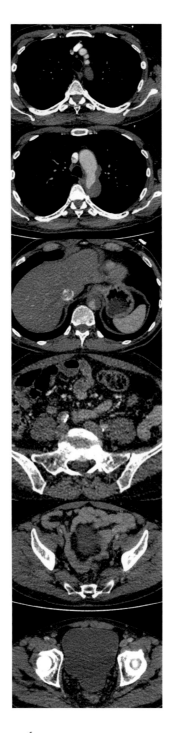

Figure 15.1 Initial CT angiogram of aorta.

The impression of the consultant vascular radiologist on-call is much the same as yours, i.e. this is a type B pattern with dissection extending down to involve the right EIA. However, the right EIA is not occluded, and there is flow into the right CFA and beyond. Given the original concerns about the right leg numbness, this would fit with the slightly compromised right EIA perfusion, but on the whole, it is deemed that his right leg would likely be ok (*there might be a dynamic obstruction here*). There is no significant renal or visceral malperfusion. The plan is for clinical assessment when the patient arrives to confirm that the right limb is not ischemic and/or threatened. Otherwise, the plan isto treat conservatively as an uncomplicated type B dissection, i.e. analgesia, BP control, HR control, ICU admission, etc.

You telephone your own ICU registrar on-call and explain that you want to transfer this patient from another hospital. You provide them with the details and they say they are happy to accept the patient, but there are currently no ICU beds available. They say the patient should go directly to A&E (*i.e. an A&E to A&E transfer*). At this point what would you do?

 A Telephone the referring A&E clinician and advise non-urgent A&E to A&E transfer.
 B Telephone the referring A&E clinician and advise urgent A&E to A&E transfer.
 C Telephone the A&E consultant on-call in your own hospital and check that they are happy to accept this patient straight into A&E as there are no ICU beds immediately available.
 D Ask the ICU registrar to sort out the transfer.
 ✓ E Telephone the A&E consultant on-call in your own hospital and check that they are happy to accept this patient straight into A&E as there are no ICU beds immediately available. Then telephone the referring A&E clinician and advise urgent A&E to A&E transfer. Then update your own vascular registrar on-call with the pertinent case details. Then document all of the above and the specific admission plan in the medical notes.

The patient arrives in A&E 35 minutes later. The vascular registrar messages you around 50 minutes later and tells you this:

> *I've just seen the patient. History is as you told me. No pain in abdomen. No chest or back pain now. Has had some decent analgesia. Diagnosed with hypertension 25 years ago but has not taken blood pressure tablets because they made him sick. He hasn't been to a GP for the past 20 years, hence no other past medical history. Smoker, around 50 pack-years. Lives with wife. Works from home. Active. End of the bed test – looks fit. BP currently is 115/77 mmHg (he is on labetalol). Heart rate 58. Sats 97% on 2 litres of oxygen. Abdomen is soft and non-tender. He has a full complement of lower limb pulses including a right DP and PT pulse. So far my impression is that there is no frank organ malperfusion and we can treat him as an uncomplicated type B dissection. ICU registrar is seeing the patient right now.*

What would you do if, upon presentation, the patient had severe abdominal pain but a completely soft abdomen?

 A Immediate laparotomy.
 ✓ B Urgent repeat CT angiogram to reassess the visceral segment and see what is going on with the SMA.
 C Immediate diagnostic laparoscopy.
 D Immediate TEVAR.
 E Increase analgesia.

What would you do if, upon presentation, the right leg was pulseless, there were sensory and motor impairment, and there was a tender right shin/calf?

✓ A Confirm the left femoral pulse was of good quality (*and at least biphasic signal using point of care ultrasound*), then proceed to a left to right femoral-femoral crossover with right leg fasciotomy.

B Commence upon intravenous heparin and keep your fingers crossed.

C Urgent repeat CT angiogram with plan likely for TEVAR followed by right iliac stenting.

D Right iliac thrombectomy.

E Right axillo-femoral bypass.

What would you do if both lower limbs were ischaemic upon presentation (Rutherford 2B)?

A Aorto-bifemoral bypass and bilateral lower limb fasciotomies.

B Left axillo-bifemoral bypass and bilateral lower limb fasciotomies.

C Right axillo-bifemoral bypass and bilateral lower limb fasciotomies.

D Urgent TEVAR.

✓ E Urgent repeat CT angiogram aorta and lower limbs, but likely then a right axillo-bifemoral bypass and bilateral lower limb fasciotomies.

If the patient had abdominal pain and raised lactate and a repeat CTA demonstrated that the dissection was now compromising the SMA origin (*but the left iliac system was still patent and the patient had a decent left femoral pulse*), what would you do?

A Urgent TEVAR and visceral branch stenting / recannalisation.

✓ B Laparotomy, inspection of the small bowel and right colon, followed by a likely left iliac to SMA bypass.

C Diagnostic laparoscopy to check that the bowel appeared to be well-perfused, and if so to proceed with TEVAR and visceral branch stenting/recannalisation in the vascular hybrid theatre.

D Laparotomy and supra-coeliac to SMA bypass.

E Laparotomy, SMA thrombectomy, retrograde SMA stenting, and bovine patch repair.

CASE REFLECTIONS

This was a fairly unexciting, completely standard type B dissection that we routinely deal with, i.e. uncomplicated and this patient was managed conservatively. However, there are two broad areas for reflection: 1) Accepting "high-stakes" referrals from outer hospitals. and 2) Having a plan for worst-case scenarios ahead of time.

1) **Accepting "high-stakes" referrals from outer hospitals.**

This is not a true description of the case. The clinician who originally referred me the patient did know that it was a type B dissection, and she had seen the patient herself. The referral itself from her was actually excellent and reflected very well on the referring clinician and the referring A&E department. However, I introduced this "referral controversy" into the equation because such a referral where the person speaking to you has not seen the patient and/or does not know the type of dissection is certainly a possibility (*and we have all received referrals like this*). I assert that one has to be pragmatic here. I do not mind accepting referrals from juniors or from someone who has not seen the patient *as long as the referral overall is of acceptable quality*. The last thing you want to do is reject a referral and insist that the referrer has to go and see the patient first, or they to get their consultant to call you directly … only to find out that the consultant who has seen the patient is dealing with a medical emergency and busy and this vascular surgery referral is actually completely justified. You can adopt this zero-tolerance approach if you want, and perhaps you are entitled to it in certain circumstances … however you have to be very careful at the same time. If you are suspected of being condescending or undermining or dismissive or obstructive or a bully then this can backfire on you big time. It would be especially bad if you were seen as a bully and you were being obstructive/awkward and the patient then had some catastrophic aortic complication because of delayed transfer, etc. My advice is to be polite over the phone, get the information you need, and do not be afraid to take a phone number and say you will call them back in a short period of time. In this case it was a completely fair referral and the referring A&E team I think actually did a really good job of working the patient up. They also sorted out an arterial line and labetolol infusion and decent analgesia prior to transferring the patient (*and I again think that was commendable*). Moral of the story is give people a chance and do not be too harsh on clinicians when they ring you up (*especially if they are junior*). Vascular surgery may not be complex to you, and the difference between a type A and type B may similarly seem straightforward to you. However, if you take a step back and see the big picture you will realise that the difference between type A and type B these days is getting more and more controversial (*i.e. the "Non-A-non-B aortic dissection" – type B dissection involving the aortic arch*).

2) **Having a plan for worst-case scenarios ahead of time.**

Aortic dissection can have many complications related to malperfusion, aneurysmal development, aortic rupture, retrograde dissection, uncontrolled blood pressure, etc. However, the ones that I particularly worry about at nighttime (i.e. when I am on-call and not many people are around) are the ones I mentioned in this case. The main ones are ipsilateral lower limb ischaemia, bilateral lower limb ischaemia and visceral malperfusion. I have a standard plan for each of these problems that has been decided ahead of time.

- Ipsilateral lower limb ischaemia = femoral – femoral crossover + fasciotomy.
- Bilateral lower limb ischaemia = right axillo-bifemoral bypass + fasciotomies.
- SMA compromise = iliac-SMA bypass.

Obviously, there are far more complex solutions to these problems and I am not saying that these are the only options available. These options may not be available of course and you might have to come up with a different solution. There may well be complex endovascular solutions that are needed and may be much better than what I am suggesting above. However, the bailout solutions I mention above will always be there at the back of my mind, and I will generally defer to these approaches if a patient is in big trouble and there is no other simpler solution available.

It is 8 pm and you are commencing your night shift on-call. A 59-year-old, poorly controlled diabetic woman is referred from A&E resus with a very nasty diabetic foot infection. Her left foot is as seen in Figure 16.1. She is pyrexial, tachycardic, and hypotensive. Her blood pressure is still low (systolic of 80 mmHg) despite 1 litre of intravenous fluids and antibiotics. The referring A&E doctor says that they cannot feel foot pulses, but can feel a femoral pulse, and possibly a weak popliteal pulse. What is your working diagnosis?

   A Necrotising fasciitis.
   B Limb-threatening neuropathic diabetic foot sepsis.
   C Life-threatening neuropathic diabetic foot sepsis.
✓ D Life-threatening neuroischaemic diabetic foot sepsis.
   E Chronic limb-threatening ischaemic with wet gangrene and soft tissue infection.

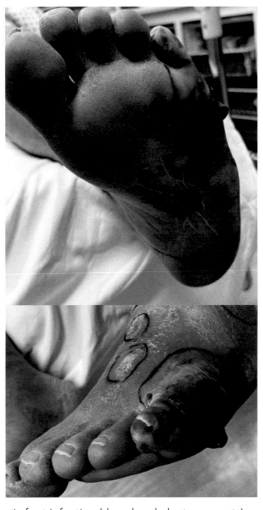

Figure 16.1   Left diabetic foot infection (dorsal and plantar aspects).

DOI: 10.1201/9781003497042-16

What do you make of the x-ray (Figure 16.2)?

✓ A Widespread gas is seen within the soft tissues surrounding the 5th metatarsal and proximal phalanx however no evidence of cortical destruction or bony resorption to suggest active osteomyelitis.

B Charcot foot changes in the midfoot.

C Gross ostemyelitic destruction of 5th metatarsal head.

D Grossly dislocated left 5th metatarsophalangeal joint.

E Gas around the 5th metatarsal head but this is simply a reflection of where an open ulcer is.

What is your overall management plan in this context?

A Intravenous antibiotics and fluids, and list for foot debridement following day.

B Urgent anaesthetic view with a view to urgent foot debridement +/− above ankle guillotine amputation the following day when medically optimised.

C Urgent anaesthetic view with a view to urgent foot debridement +/− above ankle guillotine amputation in the next few hours.

✓ D Urgent anaesthetic view with a view to urgent foot debridement +/− above ankle guillotine amputation in the next few hours, with additional referral to the intensive care team as the patient will require at least a HDU bed post-operatively.

E Urgent anaesthetic view with a view to below-knee amputation in the next few hours.

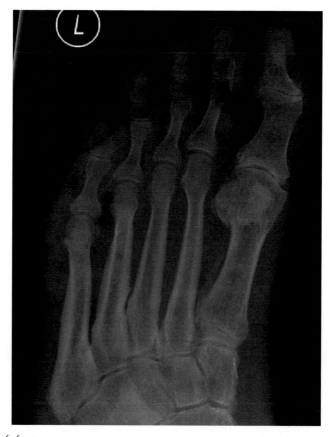

Figure 16.2   Left foot x-ray.

The theatre team say that there is a plastic surgical case that is currently booked on the emergency theatre list which needs to go first. The plastic surgical case is listed as "removal of foreign object from right buttock." This foreign object is a broken knife tip that the patient was stabbed with 24 hours ago, with the patient waiting all day for it to be removed (*but the patient is completely well with no bleeding concerns, no neurological compromise, and he is not septic*). How would you respond to this?

A Let the plastic surgeons go first. This will give you more time to optimise your patient who can go second.

✓ B Speak to the plastic surgeons and explain that your patient has a life-threatening problem and therefore vascular surgery should go first.

C Let the emergency anaesthetist decide who goes first.

D Let the plastic surgeons go first as you should not be rushing your patient to the theatre first anyway. Patients with life-threatening diabetic foot sepsis require medical optimisation first, and only when they are systemically and physiologically "well" should they proceed with surgery to achieve source control.

E Request that a second emergency theatre is opened so that vascular and plastics can both go to theatre at the same time.

The plastic surgeons are happy to let you go first because their case (*even they admit*) is not sick and can be delayed until tomorrow if necessary. The emergency theatre coordinator asks if your patient is "ready to go"? What does "ready to go" mean to you?

A Consented and marked for radical foot debridement.

B Consented and marked for radical foot debridement +/– above ankle guillotine amputation +/– proceed. Blood available (i.e. valid group and save). ECG available. Safe surgery checklist completed. Confirmed that the patient is not on any blood thinning medications. Confirmed that you have updated the ICU team in regard to need for post-op HDU bed.

✓ C Consented and marked for radical foot debridement +/– above ankle guillotine amputation +/– proceed. Blood is available (i.e. valid group and save). ECG is done. Make sure there is no metalwork in the leg at ankle level. Make sure there is no pacemaker or implantable cardiac defibrillator that needs to be turned off. Safe surgery checklist completed. Confirmed that the patient is not on any blood thinning medications. Confirmed that you have updated the ICU team in regard to need for post-op HDU bed.

D Consented and marked for radical foot debridement +/– above ankle guillotine amputation +/– proceed, blood cross-matched.

E Consented for radical foot debridement +/– proceed.

What do you see in the chest x-ray (Figure 16.3) and what is your plan?

A Normal – nil to add.

B Left basal consolidation – needs more antibiotics to target chest.

✓ C Implanted cardiac device with cardiomegaly – need to speak to cardiac electrophysiology team as this may have implications for diathermy use. Also need to be wary about giving patient too much IV fluids as it could push her into pulmonary oedema.

D Implanted cardiac device- need to speak to cardiac electrophysiology team as this may have implications for diathermy use

E Left diaphragmatic hernia – needs urgent referral to upper gastrointestinal surgeons on-call for diaphragmatic repair (*naturally prior to drainage of foot sepsis, first things must come first*).

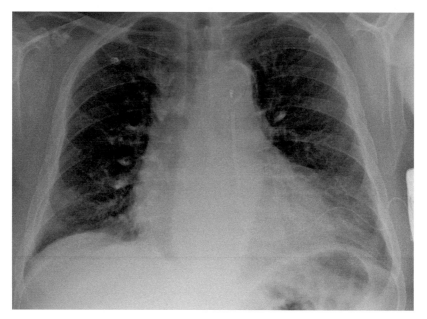

Figure 16.3 Chest x-ray.

You read through some recent cardiology letters and find this summary information: "Cardiac arrest (ventricular fibrillation) following dialysis. Subcutaneous ICD implant. Significant coronary heart disease for conservative management. Left ventricular systolic dysfunction (LV ejection fraction 40%). Mild to moderate aortic stenosis on echo. End stage renal failure secondary hypertension – on haemodialysis." You also review the blood results from today (Figure 16.4). How does this influence your overall management plan?

✓ A Anaemic, very raised inflammatory markers, clotting slightly deranged, liver tests deranged, low albumin, raised lactate, very comorbid including end-stage renal failure, heart not great … ***this patient is about as high risk as they get***. I better take things very seriously and make sure this patient gets the attention she deserves.

B Just looks a bit septic to me and she is comorbid. Just a standard diabetic foot sepsis … doesn't need to be taken too seriously. I worry more about AAA ruptures and ischaemic limbs when I am on-call.

C Yes, she is sick, but a quick foot debridement and then admission to the vascular ward for standard sepsis management is all that is needed here.

D Patient needs palliating as she is clearly end of life.

E Patient is too high-risk for surgery now, we should manage her conservatively now, and if she gets better, we can go to theatre in 48 hours time.

You go to theatre in around 1 hour. The cardiac electrophysiologist switches off the ICD (*you were informed that you are not allowed to use any form of diathermy whilst it is activated*). The anaesthetist has performed a very effective lower limb block. Is there anything else you might consider using in theatre?

A Diathermy set to kill.

✓ B Tourniquet.

C Lot of haemostatic agents.

D Loads of bone wax.

E Limit your debridement so as to limit blood loss.

Full blood Count FBC

Result	Value	Units	Ref. Range
Haemoglobin	102	g/L	135-180
White cell count	34.31	10*9/L	4.00-11.00
Platelets	358	10*9/L	150-400
Mean cell volume MCV	84	fL	78-100
Packed cell volume	0.33		0.40-0.52
Red cell count RBC	3.94	10*12/L	4.50-6.50
Mean corpusc Hb MCH	25.9	pg	27.0-32.0
RBC dist width	17.2		<15.0
Neutrophil count	30.48	10*9/L	2.00-7.50
Lymphocyte count	1.33	10*9/L	1.00-4.50
Monocyte count	1.76	10*9/L	0.20-0.80
Eosinophil count	0.05	10*9/L	0.04-0.40
Basophil count	0.09	10*9/L	<0.10
Large unstained cell	0.61	10*9/L	<0.60
% Hypochromic cells	29	%	
Set Comment:	Neutrophil leucocytosis. Suggest mo		

Clotting Screen

Result	Value	Units	Ref. Range
Prothrombin time	17	s	9-14
INR (p=poc)	1.4		
APTT (a=anticoag therapy)	35.8	s	23.5-37.5
APTT Ratio (a=anticoag therapy)	1.2		0.8-1.2
Set Comment:			

Calcium-adj,Alb,PO4

Result	Value	Units	Ref. Range
Calcium-adjusted	2.66	mmol/L	2.20-2.60
Albumin	19	g/L	35-50
Phosphate	1.29	mmol/L	0.80-1.50
Alk Phos	259	iu/L	30-130
Set Comment:	Please Note: Adjusted calcium calcu		

CRP

Result	Value	Units	Ref. Range
CRP	365	mg/L	<10.0
Set Comment:			

Liver Function Test

Result	Value	Units	Ref. Range
Bilirubin	8	umol/L	2-21
ALT	73	iu/L	<40
Albumin	19	g/L	35-50
Alk Phos	259	iu/L	30-130
Set Comment:			

Urea & Electrolytes

Result	Value	Units	Ref. Rang
Sodium	134	mmol/L	133-146
Potassium	4.9	mmol/L	3.5-5.3
Urea	16.6	mmol/L	2.5-7.8
Creatinine	602	umol/L	64-104
eGFR	8	mL/min/1.73m2	

ACID/BASE 37.0°C
pH 7.35
pCO_2 5.98 kPa
pO_2 4.87 kPa
HCO_3 act 24.6 mmol/l
HCO_3 std 23.1 mmol/l
BE(B) 1.0 mmol/l

CO-OXIMETRY
tHb 109 g/l
FO_2Hb 68.3 %
FCOHb 0.7 %
FMetHb 0.0 %
FHHb 31.0 %

ELECTROLYTES
Na+ 130.1 mmol/l
K+ 4.65 mmol/l
Ca++ 1.31 mmol/l
Cl- 94 mmol/l

METABOLITES
Glu 11.8 mmol/l
Lac 2.39 mmol/l

Figure 16.4 Blood results and venous blood gas.

Vascular Surgery

The patient is on the table with an above-knee tourniquet applied. What is your surgical approach?

✓ A Start with a foot debridement to confirm how bad the sepsis is. If the sepsis is not as bad as expected, proceed with an attempt at limb salvage. If the sepsis is as bad as expected, have a low threshold to convert to immediate above ankle guillotine amputation.
B Proceed with an immediate above ankle guillotine amputation.
C Proceed with an immediate below-knee amputation.
D Just do a 5th ray amputation and leave the foot open to drain further. The patient can come back for further debridement surgery if she continues to be septic at wound review in 48 hours.
E Proceed with an immediate above-knee amputation.

You initially commence with a 5th ray amputation. You see necrosis and pus invading the 4th metatarsophalangeal joint. You proceed to incision down the medial border of the 4th toe, and find there is necrosis and pus invading the 3rd metatarsophalangeal joint. You make an incision down the dorsum of the foot and see there is pus around the extensor tendons. You make an incision down the plantar aspect of the foot curving towards the medial aspect (Loeffler Ballard incision) – again there is pus in the foot and the tendon sheaths are infected. You make another incision down the medial border of the 2nd toe and there is smelly necrotic tissue invading around this region also. The septic process has clearly compromised the dorum and plantar aspect of the foot down to the midfoot level, and it is almost reaching the hindfoot. The sepsis has not crossed the ankle joint however. What are you going to do now?

A Left forefoot amputation.
B Left ankle disarticulation.
✓ C Left above ankle guillotine amputation.
D Left 2nd to 5th ray amputations.
E Left below-knee amputation.

The patient proceeds with a guillotine amputation above the ankle (*see Figure 16.5*). What would be your post-operative plan now?

A High observation ward admission with a view to intravenous antibiotics, cautious intravenous fluid replacement, and once medically optimised for a formal below-knee amputation (*at a later date*).
B Vascular ward admission with a view to intravenous antibiotics, cautious intravenous fluid replacement, and an above-knee amputation the following day when medically optimised.
C HDU admission with a view to intravenous antibiotics, cautious intravenous fluid replacement, renal replacement therapy, inotropic support for his septic shock, and once medically optimised for a formal below-knee amputation (*at a later date*).
D Transfer to the diabetic ward for optimisation of diabetic control and plan for a formal below-knee amputation in 3 months when her diabetic control is perfect (*her HBA1c is 80*).
✓ E HDU admission with a view to intravenous antibiotics, variable rate insulin infusion, very cautious intravenous fluid replacement, arrange dialysis for following morning, inotropic support for septic shock, and once medically optimised for a formal below-knee amputation (at a later date).

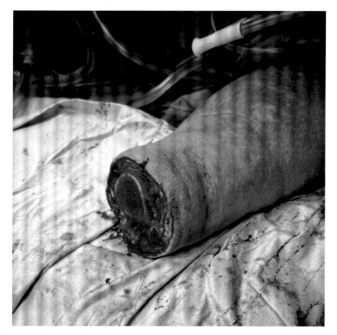

Figure 16.5   Above ankle guillotine amputation.

CASE REFLECTIONS

Vascular surgery is complex and covers a very large area, from acute limb ischaemia to ruptured aneurysms to carotid disease to renal access to trauma … but in my opinion diabetic foot disease is the disease entity that is the most complex, the most challenging, and the most risky.

It is so easy to underestimate diabetic foot sepsis. It is so easy to view such as cases as nothing more than a quick toe amputation followed by a crural angioplasty. I wish they were all so simple. However, I find that whenever I have to do an emergency guillotine amputation out of hours in this context, the patient is almost always frail, very comorbid (*often with cardiac/respiratory/renal impairment*), has peripheral arterial disease, and is in septic shock. The guillotine amputation may be an "easy operation," but this doesn't change the fact that the patient is still incredibly sick and very high risk.

My advice to you would be to take these sorts of patients extremely seriously. Be thorough with your clinical assessments. Try to avoid excessive delays getting into theatre for source control. Make pragmatic decisions i.e. if the foot looks awful and it is *life-threatening* foot sepsis then have a low threshold to convert to an above ankle guillotine amputation. If you are not going to guillotine the patient and want to try and achieve limb salvage then make sure you have genuinely cleared the foot sepsis. Get the intensive care team involved early. Have a low threshold to involve other specialities such as diabetes, renal, and cardiology. Make sure they get the right antibiotics (*get microbiology involved in you are in any doubt*). Don't rush into doing a formal below-knee amputation until they are truly medically optimised. Make sure you document things clearly in the medical notes. Do things by the book.

CASE 17: RENAL ACCESS

A 62-year-old diabetic woman presents to your renal access outpatient clinic being considered for a fistula creation. She has end stage renal failure with an eGFR of 11% and has opted for haemodialysis. She is right handed. She also had a background of lower limb peripheral arterial disease that is being managed conservatively (*she has intermittent calf claudication bilaterally*). She has already had her fistula planning ultrasound, but the patient only agreed to have her left arm scanned. Please review the fistula ultrasound results (Figure 17.1), and indicate what you think is the most appropriate renal access option for her.

   A Left radiocephalic fistula creation.
✓ B Left brachiocephalic fistula creation.
   C Left basilic vein transposition.
   D Left brachio-axillary graft.
   E Left brachio-basilic forearm loop graft.

The patient agrees to go ahead with a left brachiocephalic fistula creation under local anaesthetic as a day-case procedure. What risks would you consent this patient for?

   A Bleeding, infection, neurovascular injury, scarring, steal syndrome, ischaemic mono-melic neuropathy, fistula failure, need for further procedures, local anaesthetic risks.
   B Bleeding, infection, neurovascular injury, scarring, steal syndrome, fistula failure, need for further procedures, local anaesthetic risks.
   C Bleeding, infection, neurovascular injury, scarring, failure to mature, fistula failure, need for further procedures, local anaesthetic risks.
   D Bleeding, infection, neurovascular injury, scarring, steal syndrome, ischaemic mono-melic neuropathy, failure to mature, fistula failure, need for further procedures, local anaesthetic risks.
✓ E Bleeding, infection, neurovascular injury, scarring, steal syndrome, ischaemic mono-melic neuropathy, failure to mature, fistula failure, aneurysmal development, need for further procedures, anaesthetic risks, and medical complications such as MI, DVT/PE, chest infection.

The patient is offered a block by the anaesthetist, but she would actually prefer a local anaesthetic approach. You therefore inject local anaesthetic under ultrasound guidance into the antecubital fossa and proceed with surgery. What would be your preferred incision for creating this brachiocephalic fistula?

   A Vertical incision in the antecubital fossa.
   B Lazy S incision in the antecubital fossa.
   C Horizontal incision in the antecubital fossa.
✓ D Lazy S or horizontal incision in the antecubital fossa with pre-marked brachial artery and cephalic vein (*using ultrasound*).
   E Upside-down smiley face incision in the antecubital fossa.

During dissection of the brachial artery, you accidentally injure the brachial vein and it starts bleeding. How would you manage this?

   A Panic and start applying blind monopolar diathermy to the bleeding area.
✓ B Stay calm and apply gentle pressure with a dry swab for 2 minutes, then lift up and see if it is still bleeding.
   C Throw some big under-running 3–0 vicryl sutures to the area of bleeding.
   D Apply a clip above and below the bleeding area and then simply ligate the brachial vein.
   E Apply a load of haemostatic agents to the area and carry on with the operation.

DOI: 10.1201/9781003497042-17

Left Upper limb Artery Mapping

Brachial artery distal = 4.6 mm
Radial artery mid = 1.9 mm
Radial artery distal = 1.6 mm

Left Upper limb Vein Mapping

Tourniquet applied:

Cephalic vein distal humerus = 4.6 mm

Cephalic vein mid forearm = 1.8 mm
Cephalic vein distal forearm = 1.9 mm

Basilic vein distal humerus = 2.9 mm

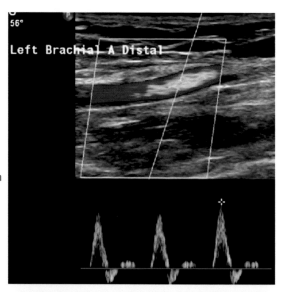

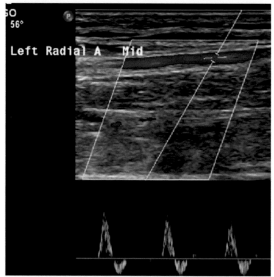

Figure 17.1 Fistula mapping ultrasound for the left arm in a patient fast-approaching the need for haemodialysis.

After applying gentle pressure with a dry swab for 2 minutes you lift it up and find that the bleeding has stopped. You then dissect out the brachial artery and sloop it proximally and distally. You then disconnect the cephalic vein distally and distend it with some heparinised saline. You do a longitudinal arteriotomy into the brachial artery and proceed to perform an end to side anastomosis using 6-0 Prolene. Upon release of the fistula there is an excellent thrill, but you cannot feel a pulse in the brachial artery beyond the anastomosis. You also cannot feel a radial pulse. You ask for the handheld Doppler and can barely hear any signal in the brachial artery beyond your anastomosis. What would you do now?

A Accept this result as the patient has a good thrill in the fistula. The hand will likely survive on collaterals.

B Ligate the fistula as clearly the patient has a significant steal syndrome.

✓ C Take the anastomosis down and proceed to a brachial embolectomy, then re-do your fistula anastomosis.

    D Take the anastomosis down and proceed to a brachial to radial artery bypass using reversed great saphenous vein.

    E Make an arteriotomy in the fistula hood and perform on-table thrombolysis down the brachial, radial, and ulnar arteries.

After taking your anastomosis down to proceed with a brachial embolectomy you find that one of your anastomotic stitches had actually caught the posterior wall of the brachial artery and had completely occluded any flow distally. The brachial artery is now back bleeding tremendously so you decide not to perform an embolectomy. You re-do the fistula anastomosis again. This time there is still an excellent thrill in the fistula, but also a good distal brachial and radial pulse and the hand pinks up rapidly. You complete the wound closure and the patient goes into theatre recovery.

Thirty minutes later you are called urgently into recovery because the patient is complaining of severe pain in the ipsilateral forearm and hand. There is an excellent thrill in the fistula. There is no bleeding and no haematoma. There is a bounding radial pulse. The hand is well perfused. The patient has paraesthesia of the forearm and hand, and she has reduced power in the hand. What is your working diagnosis?

    A Acute limb ischaemia.

    B Steal syndrome.

    C Stroke.

  ✓ D Ischaemic monomelic neuropathy.

    E Local anaesthetic complication (*i.e. you must have compromised the median and ulnar nerves*).

What would be your immediate management plan?

    A Improved analgesia and anaesthetic referral for a supraclavicular block.

    B Urgent CT angiogram.

    C Urgent CT brain.

  ✓ D Immediate return to theatre for fistula ligation.

    E Allow 6 hours to see if her symptoms improve. If not, then return to theatre for fistula ligation.

You take the patient back to theatre and ligate the fistula. Her neurological symptoms rapidly improve. On table the patient asks if you can create a fistula in the contralateral arm as she is approaching the need for dialysis very soon. What would you do in this context?

    A Start performing an ultrasound assessment of the right arm. If she has a simple fistula option proceed with something like a radiocephalic or brachiocephalic fistula creation.

    B Perform an ultrasound assessment of the right arm in theatre. Decide upon an appropriate fistula right now, and plan to bring her back the following week for another fistula creation.

  ✓ C Inform the patient that now is simply not the right time to be thinking of fistula planning or fistula creation in the other arm. She has just had a major complication and rushing into another fistula creation on the other side is unwise. She should recover from this episode first and then come back to the next available access clinic to discuss further access options.

    D Ask the anaesthetist to put the patient to sleep and then proceed immediately with a peritoneal dialysis tube insertion.

    E Ask the renal consultant on-call to come to theatre and insert a tunnelled neck line.

After ligating the fistula, the patient returns to theatre recovery again. Twenty minutes later, you are asked to see her urgently again because she has a sizeable haematoma in the left antecubital fossa. The haematoma is expanding in front of your eyes. What are you going to do now?

  A Pressure dressing and reassess in 1 hour.
  ✓ B Take back to theatre (*again*) for haemorrhage control. This is likely bleeding from the brachial artery arteriotomy site (*i.e. suture line bleeding*).
  C Urgent referral to interventional radiology for a brachial artery covered stent insertion.
  D Give the patient tranexamic acid and apply a pressure dressing.
  E Open the wound in recovery and oversew any bleeding venous structures.

One week later, the patient re-presents to A&E with a slightly tender and very minor swelling in the left antecubital fossa. There is minor erythema around the incision site and the patient has a WBC of 12 and a CRP of 47. The patient is systemically well and apyrexial. She is not reporting any further bleeding from the wound. She has an intact radial pulse. An ultrasound reveals a very small haematoma underneath the skin but no pseudoaneurysm. What is your diagnosis and management plan?

  A Infected haematoma and/or cellulitis. For oral antibiotics and close outpatient follow-up.
  ✓ B Likely wound cellulitis for oral antibiotics and close outpatient follow-up.
  C Infected haematoma that requires urgent admission for intravenous antibiotics and formal surgical washout.
  D Wound cellulitis that requires urgent admission for intravenous antibiotics.
  E Infected fistula anastomosis that is clearly still bleeding and requires an urgent trip back to the theatre.

One day later the patient returns to A&E out of hours with severe sepsis. She now has erythema spreading up and down the arm. You can feel crepitus under her skin and there is skin blistering as well. A CT angiogram has ruled out a pseudoaneurysm but there is gas in the soft tissues. Her WBC is 35 and her CRP is 389. She is pyrexic and tachycardic and hypotensive. Her arterial blood gas reveals a pH of 7.24 and a lactate of 5. What is your diagnosis?

  A Severely infected haematoma.
  B Severe cellulitis.
  C Compartment syndrome.
  D Steal syndrome.
  ✓ E Necrotising soft tissue infection.

CASE REFLECTIONS

This is not a real case, but again one that deliberately contains an "orgy" of complications and challenges for educational purposes. There is one area I wish to focus upon here – **THE 1% AND THE ROLLERCOASTER**.

Whenever you see a vascular surgery patient on the ward or in the outpatient department, you always speak to them and talk about the proposed procedure, and you mention a legion of potential risks. In the case of a lower limb angioplasty, for example, you might say something like this:

> *This procedure involves a femoral artery puncture in the groin, shooting down x-ray dye down the leg to visualise the artery, passing a wire through any narrowings and then doing either balloon stretching or stenting. The reason we are doing it is to make*

the blood supply to your leg better to relieve your pain, help that ulcer to heal, and/or to possibly make your walking distance improve. There are risks however which include femoral access complications i.e. a small risk of needing to go to theatre to repair the femoral artery in the groin, a small risk of making the blood supply to your leg worse, the need for further procedures in case of a complication, a small risk of a major amputation, a small risk of making your kidneys worse and you possibly needing to go on dialysis, a risk of severe allergic reaction to the x-ray dye, etc. However, most of the time these complications do not take place, so don't be too alarmed. We have to mention these risks, and we mention them to everyone going for this procedure.

It is likely in such a context a patient would agree to the procedure, and the procedure would be a success, and the patient would be happy with the result. This is probably the majority of outcomes within this context. However, there will always be that one person in a hundred (*the 1%*) who unfortunately experiences the negative outcome/s. That patient may have a femoral artery bleed, require an emergency bovine patch repair, the bovine patch then gets infected and blows, then the patient ends up with an above-knee amputation. The same patient may also end up in renal failure and die. This is an extreme fictional example but I have definitely seen things like this happen. The *1% AND THE ROLLERCOASTER* is, therefore, a real phenomenon in vascular surgery. It relates to endovascular surgery, carotid surgery, renal access surgery, aortic surgery, etc.

The reason I mention this is because it is all about *surgical decision-making, patient counselling, and informed consent*. If you have a patient with life-limiting intermittent claudication with a minor SFA stenosis who is still smoking and not on the best medical therapy and you refer them for a "straightforward" day-case SFA angioplasty, it could very well be this patient who represents the 1% (*with an above-knee amputation and secondary type 2 myocardial infarction ensuing*). If you have a female patient with a borderline carotid stenosis and a TIA 2 months ago and she has had no further neurological events since being commenced on best medical therapy, well you could proceed with a carotid endarterectomy but again she could represent the 1% (*and end up with a dense paraplegia and a cranial nerve injury*). If you have a female patient on oestrogen hormone replacement therapy and a body mass index of 39 who turns up for right GSV endovenous ablation because of C2 varicose veins and you decide to proceed on the day, she could very well be that 1% who ends up getting a saddle pulmonary embolus and dying 3 days later in A&E resus after an unsuccessful thrombolysis attempt.

The point I am making is that if you are going to take risks (*which vascular surgery is frankly all about*) you should be cognisant of the *1% AND THE ROLLERCOASTER* hiding in the background. Imagine that the patient in front of you could very well be that 1%, and if you operate on them you may find yourself on that rollercoaster. If the patient has been thoroughly counselled and consented, if the indication is sound and the benefits of proceeding appear to outweigh the risks, then it is probably fair game to proceed. However, if the patient does not really know what they are signing up for, if the consent form is missing various important risks, and the indication for the procedure is dubious, you are potentially walking on very thin ice.

INDEX

Index

For Product Safety Concerns and Information please contact our
EU representative GPSR@taylorandfrancis.com Taylor & Francis
Verlag GmbH, Kaufingerstraße 24, 80331 München, Germany